Practical
Evaluation and Management
Coding

T0211782

CURRENT ◊ CLINICAL ◊ PRACTICE

NEIL S. SKOLNIK, MD • SERIES EDITOR

Anxiety Disorders: A Pocket Guide for Primary Care, edited by JOHN R. VANIN AND JAMES D. HELSLEY, 2008

Practical Evaluation and Management Coding: A Four-Step Guide for Physicians and Coders, by CHRISTOPHER L. TAYLOR, 2007

Women's Health in Clinical Practice: A Handbook for Primary Care, edited by AMY LYNN CLOUSE AND KATHERINE SHERIF, 2008

Primary Care Sleep Medicine: A Practical Guide, edited by J. F. PAGEL AND S. R. PANDI-PERUMAL, 2008

Essential Practice Guidelines in Primary Care, edited by NEIL S. SKOLNIK, 2007

Sexually Transmitted Diseases: A Practical Guide for Primary Care, edited by ANITA NELSON AND JOANN WOODWARD, 2007

Allergic Diseases: Diagnosis and Treatment, Third Edition, edited by PHIL LIEBERMAN AND JOHN A. ANDERSON, 2007

Headache and Chronic Pain Syndromes: The Case-Based Guide to Targeted Assessment and Treatment, DAWN A. MARCUS, 2007

Bone Densitometry in Growing Patients: Guidelines for Clinical Practice, edited by AENOR J. SAWYER, LAURA K. BACHRACH, AND ELLEN B. FUNG, 2007

The Handbook of Contraception: A Guide for Practical Management, edited by DONNA SHOUPE AND SIRI L. KJOS, 2006

Obstetrics in Family Medicine: A Practical Guide, PAUL LYONS, 2006

Psychiatric Disorders in Pregnancy and the Postpartum: Principles and Treatment, edited by VICTORIA HENDRICK, 2006

Disorders of the Respiratory Tract: Common Challenges in Primary Care, edited by MATTHEW L. MINTZ, 2006

Cardiology in Family Practice: A Practical Guide, STEVEN M. HOLLENBERG AND TRACY WALKER, 2006

Bronchial Asthma: A Guide for Practical Understanding and Treatment, Fifth Edition, edited by M. ERIC GERSHWIN AND TIMOTHY E. ALBERTSON, 2006

Dermatology Skills for Primary Care: An Illustrated Guide, DANIEL J. TROZAK, DAN J. TENNENHOUSE, AND JOHN J. RUSSELL, 2006

Thyroid Disease: A Case-Based and Practical Guide for Primary Care, EMANUEL O. BRAMS, 2005

Type 2 Diabetes, Pre-Diabetes, and the Metabolic Syndrome: The Primary Care Guide to Diagnosis and Management, RONALD A. CODARIO, 2005

Chronic Pain: A Primary Care Guide to Practical Management, DAWN A. MARCUS, 2005

Bone Densitometry in Clinical Practice: Application and Interpretation, Second Edition, SYDNEY LOU BONNICK, 2004

Cancer Screening: A Practical Guide for Physicians, edited by KHALID AZIZ AND GEORGE Y. WU, 2001

Hypertension Medicine, edited by MICHAEL A. WEBER, 2001

Allergic Diseases: Diagnosis and Treatment, Second Edition, edited by PHIL LIEBERMAN AND JOHN A. ANDERSON, 2000

Parkinson's Disease and Movement Disorders: Diagnosis and Treatment Guidelines for the Practicing Physician, edited by CHARLES H. ADLER AND J. ERIC AHLSKOG, 2000

Bone Densitometry in Clinical Practice: Application and Interpretation, SYDNEY LOU BONNICK, 1998

Practical Evaluation and Management Coding

A Four-Step Guide
for Physicians and Coders

Christopher L. Taylor, MD

Departments of Neurosurgery and Radiology
University of New Mexico Medical School
Albuquerque, NM

HUMANA PRESS ✳ TOTOWA, NEW JERSEY

© 2007 Humana Press Inc., a part of Springer Science+Business Media, LLC
999 Riverview Drive, Suite 208
Totowa, New Jersey, 07512
www.humanapress.com

All rights reserved. No part of this book may be reproduced, stored in a retrevial system, or transmitted in any form or by any means, electronic, mechanical, photocopying, microfilming, recording, or otherwise without written permission from the Publisher.

All articles, comments, opinions, conclusions, or recommendations, are those of the author(s), and do not necessarily relfect the views of the publisher.

Due diligence has been taken by the publisher, editors, and authors of this book to assure the accuracy of the information published and to describe generally accepted practices. The contributors herein have carefully checked to ensure that the drug selection and dosages set forth in this text are accurate and in accord with the standards accepted at the time of publication. Notwithstanding, as new research, changes in government regulations, and knowledge from clinical experience relating to drug therapy and drug reactions constantly occurs, the reader is advised to check the product information provided by the manufacturer of each drug for any change in dosages or for additional warnings and contraindications. This is of utmost importance when the recommended drug herein is a new or infrequently used drug. It is the responsibility of the treating physican to determine dosages and treatment strategies for individual patients. Futher it is the responsibility of the health care provider to ascertain the Food and Drug Administration status of each drug or device used in their clinical pratice. The publisher, editors, and authors are not responsible for errors or omissions or for any consequences from the application of the information presented in this book and make no warranty, express or implied, with respect to the contents in this publication.

Cover design by Karen Schulz

This publication is printed on acid-free paper. ∞

For additional copies, pricing for bulk purchases, and/or information about other Humana titles, contact Humana at the above address or at any of the following numbers: Tel.:973-256-1699; Fax: 973-256-83411; or visit our Website: http://www.humanapress.com.

Photocopy Authorization Policy:
Authorization to photocopy items for internal or personal use, or the internal or personal use of specific clients, is granted by Humana Press Inc., provided that the base fee of US $30.00 per copy is paid directly to the Copyright Clearance Center at 222 Rosewood Drive, Danvers, MA 01923. For those organizations that have been granted a photocopy license from the CCC, a separate system of payment has been arranged and is acceptable to Humana Press Inc. The fee code for users of the Transcriptional Reporting Service is: [978-1-58829-694-8/07 $30.00]

10 9 8 7 6 5 4 3 2 1

ISBN 978-1-59745-314-1 (eBook)

Library of Congress Control Number: 2007922049

Series Editor's Introduction

Practical Evaluation and Management Coding by Christopher Taylor, MD, is a practical handbook about an aspect of medical practice that continues to be a challenge to many physicians—correct coding. The coding system for Evaluation and Management services is complex, yet essential for physicians to master in order to bill for and receive correct payment for their services to patients. Dr. Taylor reviews the rationale for the coding system, and then gives a systematic yet simple explanation of how the system works and how to determine the proper code for each visit. His explanations are clear and concise.

This insightful book can lead to an understanding of coding—and its correct application, and can serve as an excellent reference when questions arise.

Practical Evaluation and Management Coding is one of those rare books that has a place on every physician's shelf.

Neil Skolnik, MD
Associate Director
Family Medicine Residency
Abington Memorial Hospital
Professor of Family and Community Medicine
Temple University School of Medicine

Preface

Duke Samson is the world's greatest cerebrovascular surgeon and everything that I know about CPT coding I learned from him. Indirectly.

During my fellowship in Dr. Samson's department I was surprised by the attention paid to the details of proper coding. Surgeries were reviewed weekly by our coders and surgeons, and Dr. Samson required everyone in the department to devote an entire day annually to reviewing the latest changes in CPT codes. Prior to this, through my entire residency, I had only a vague notion of what a CPT code was. But now the message was clear: this is important. However, after three years I realized that while I could code surgeries accurately I still did not understand evaluation and management (E/M) codes. I was determined to understand this arcane subject. My method of making simple (or at least understandable) a ridiculously complex set of algorithms is the subject of this book.

The entire book is supposed to be a shortcut to understanding, but here is the shortcut to the book: medical decision making. Medical decision making is the key to proper E/M coding. If you determine your medical decision making first, the history and physical will follow naturally. If you understand the medical decision making of an encounter, everything else will fit easily into place.

Christopher L. Taylor

Contents

Series Editor's Introduction by *Neil Skolnik* v

Preface vii

Introduction 1

Step 1
Identify the Patient Category 9

Step 2
Use the Medical Decision-Making Table 15

Step 3
Select the Appropriate Level for History
and Examination 25

Step 4
Identify the Correct CPT Code and Modifier 43

Appendices 49
A: E/M Coding Guide 51
B: New Patient Consultation Template:
   Neurosurgical Practice 55
C: New Patient Consultation Template:
   Low Back Pain 61

D: 1997 Documentation Guidelines for Evaluation
   and Management Services   65
E: Other Resources for Coding Information   115
F: A Detailed Analysis of Two Coding Methods
   Summarized in the Introduction   117

Index   121

Introduction

For better or worse, physicians in the United States are not paid for their work in the same way as are most other service professionals. Your attorney will talk to you in the office, send you a bill based on the number of minutes spent with you, and expect to receive payment for his or her services. Your accountant will collect your financial documents, prepare your tax returns, and send you a bill that reflects the complexity of your financial situation. Again, he or she will expect to receive payment in full for the services provided. Physicians, however, receive most of the payment for their services from third-party insurers based on rates that are predetermined by the government (for Medicare and Medicaid) or by the insurer. In this respect, running a medical practice has much more in common with operating an auto body repair shop than it does with other professions.

Physicians commonly serve patients who have health insurance through the Centers for Medicare and Medicaid Services (CMS) or through a private health insurance company. When a service is rendered to a person who is covered by one of these entities, the physician then identifies that service by a numeric code. The code is submitted to the insurer, and the insurer pays the physician based on its standard reimbursement rate for that code. Reimbursement rates, or "fee schedules," for private health insurers are agreed to by contract between the insurer and the physician. The fee schedule used by CMS is set by the U.S. Congress.

Whether a generalist or specialist, procedurally oriented or not, the most common service a clinical physician provides is the outpatient office visit. In addition, most doctors in clinical practice will see patients in the hospital. Specialists with training beyond general medicine or pediatrics will also provide consultations, either in the office or in the hospital. A simple, logical method of determining the correct numeric code for each of these services is the main topic of this book.

Current Procedural Terminology (CPT) is a set of numeric codes developed and copyrighted by the American Medical Association (AMA) to describe all of the medical services and procedures that physicians provide. The 2005 edition of CPT runs more than 500 pages and covers everything from "Anesthesia for procedures on salivary glands . . . (00100)" to "Home infusion/ specialty drug administration . . . (99601)." Evaluation and management (E/M) is a section of CPT that includes all of the codes designated for describing office visits, hospital visits, and consultations. These are the most commonly used codes for office-based physicians in clinical practice.

For any given patient encounter, the correct CPT code is determined by a finite set of variables. All of these variables are defined by CPT and, with one exception, are easily learned even if not exactly self-evident. The exception for most of the codes discussed in this text is the "level of service." For many of these codes, the fifth digit will range from 1 to 5 (1 to 3 in some cases) denoting lower or higher levels of service. A "level 1" code will indicate a relatively simple service and, therefore, will receive relatively low compensation. A "level 5" code indicates the most difficult cases and receives the highest compensation.

The accuracy with which E/M codes are applied is of great importance to both the physician who submits them and to the insurer who writes the check to reimburse his or her services. If the submitted code reflects a lower level of service than was provided, then the physician will not receive all of the compensation to which he or she is entitled under the current CMS fee schedule or under the contract with the insurance carrier. If the submitted code reflects a higher level of service than was provided, then the insurer (or the government) will spend money unnecessarily. Whether intentional or not, "up-coding" may be considered fraud and can expose the practitioner to monetary penalties and risk of prosecution. U.S. taxpayers spent $309 billion on Medicare in 2004. Of that total, $54 billion dollars went to physician fee schedule services (2005 Annual Report of the Boards of Trustees of the Federal Hospital Insurance and Federal Supplementary Medical Insurance Trust Funds). Those services included E/M, as well as other more costly items, including surgical fees, invasive diagnostic procedures, professional fees for radiological services, and so on. Nevertheless, the absolute dollar amount spent on health care is staggering.

Correct coding is also crucial to the bottom line of a successful medical practice. As an example, consider two primary care physicians, each in solo practice (Table I.1). Both physicians saw an average of 110 patients each week in 2004. Allowing 4 weeks for vacation, each doctor produced 5,280 patient visits that year. Now compare their coding strategies. Dr. Average chose to code all encounters at the average level for a patient who had previously received care. Revenue from CMS for E/M services for the year totaled $277,989. Dr. Correct makes the effort to code correctly. Dr. Correct recognized that 25% of his patients were new to the practice and that some of these were complex cases. He also identified 20% of his patients as having had follow-up visits that were less complicated than average. By coding these office visits

Table I.1 Comparison of coding methods.

	Dr. Average	Dr. Correct	2004 Survey of General Practitioners
Number of patients seen per week	110	110	110
Coding method	One-size-fits-all	Correct	?
Gross revenue	$208,494	$390,956	$260,000

correctly, Dr. Correct had revenue for E/M services for the year totaling $390,959. Compare these numbers to the actual average 2004 practice revenue for general practitioners of $260,000. Of course, the numbers in this example are not directly comparable to the real results of physicians in practice because of several necessary assumptions. However, the numbers do give a valid indication of the effect that correct coding can have on the financial health of a medical practice. (A detailed explanation of this analysis and references are shown in Appendix F.)

As illustrated in this example, correct coding for E/M services has two significant advantages for a medical practice. As anyone trying to sell their seminar, training program, or book on correct coding will tell you, changing from a one-size-fits-all method of applying CPT codes to correct coding can mean more dollars coming in to your practice. The second benefit, often overlooked but no less important, is that learning to apply CPT codes correctly is both an ethical way to do business and a powerful means of decreasing your liability in the event of an audit by CMS or a review by one of the insurance carriers with whom a physician has a contract.

It should be an easy task for a practicing physician to choose a code that accurately reflects the amount of effort expended and complexity of care for a patient encounter. Any doctor who has kept regular office hours for more than a few months knows the difference between a routine case and one that represents a complex medical problem. In fact, for some specialists, a routine day in the clinic may include several patients with the same chief complaint all of whom require essentially the same diagnostic workup and therapeutic management. However, despite this intuitive understanding of the relative simplicity or complexity of each patient visit, payers—specifically CMS—require objective guidelines for evaluating the level of service provided. This should not be surprising given the amount of money spent on E/M services by CMS and private insurers. The most recent set of guidelines issued by CMS is the 1997 Documentation Guidelines for Evaluation and Management Services, which is reprinted in its entirety in Appendix D.

It must be noted at this point that complete documentation of every component of each patient encounter is essential. It is axiomatic in our current medical-legal environment that "if it wasn't documented, it wasn't done." Whether true or not, the principal of complete documentation should be a fundamental component of your billing method. The chapters of this text will describe the necessary components for the most common E/M codes. It is assumed that the reader not only meets the criteria for use of a certain code, but that he or she also documents the fact that they have done so. With the proliferation of electronic medical records (EMR), it should become easier to ensure that documentation meets standards for a given code. However, even if EMR is not used, dictation templates may be created for common presenting complaints that meet coding guidelines for various common presentations. Examples of dictation templates used in my practice for new patients (with neurological complaints unrelated to spinal column disease) and for new patients with low-back pain are shown in Appendices B and C.

The next four chapters detail a simple, step-by-step approach to determining the correct CPT code for the most common patient encounters—outpatient and hospital patient visits and consultations. Step 1, identify the patient category, is straightforward and requires only that the physician learn a few definitions and follow what is essentially a decision tree described in words. After completing Step 1, the physician will have the first four digits of the correct five-digit code. Steps 2, 3, and 4 deal with the components of E/M coding that most closely resemble the "history and physical" as taught in medical school. The SOAP (subjective information, objective information, assessment, plan) method of clinical practice is translated into the vernacular of the 1997 CMS Guidelines and becomes "history, examination, and medical decision making." Step 2, use the medical decision-making table, is where, I believe, this text makes the most important contribution to simple, correct, and logical E/M coding. As detailed in that chapter, determining the correct code for E/M services is done logically and simply if the physician reverses years of training and works backward, first determining the level of medical decision making and second determining the appropriate history and examination. Step 3, select the appropriate level for history and examination, requires referencing the 1997 CMS Guidelines to ensure that certain minimum levels of evaluation are performed. Step 4, identify the correct CPT code and modifier, requires only that you take information from Steps 2 and 3 and compare it to a table of available codes. At each step, the physician is encouraged to refer to the E/M Coding Guide that is shown in Appendix A. The E/M Coding Guide is a logically organized worksheet for determining proper CPT coding.

It is not my goal or my practice to bill every new patient encounter at the highest reimbursing level 5 code. Rather, my intention is to quickly and correctly identify the appropriate code for the many repetitive patient encounters that are a daily routine of clinical medicine. If a physician decides that every patient that complains of coughing requires a chest X-ray and laboratory testing and is at risk of death because of the possibility of antibiotic-resistant pneumonia, the physician may choose to code each of them as a level 5 visit. The physician may even meet the documentation requirements for this level of code to the letter. Whether or not the practice is ethical and justified will be left to each physician to decide and, possibly at some time in your career, by external auditors.

My approach to E/M coding is an attempt to apply the guidelines set forth by CMS logically. While I have made every effort within this text to conform to the definitions and standards set forth by CMS and AMA, the publications of CMS and AMA are the only authoritative works on this subject.

This text is primarily concerned with accurate coding of E/M encounters and not with anticipated, actual, or appropriate reimbursement for these services. I will, however, occasionally make comments regarding the relative value units (RVU) assigned to certain codes by CMS. RVU, as determined by CMS, are published on its website. If multiplied by the current conversion factor specific to a physician's geographic location, it is possible to determine the expected reimbursement from CMS for each of these services. Therefore, for services provided to a patient covered by CMS, RVU are directly correlated with reimbursement. This is not necessarily true for other third-party payers. While some insurers reimburse a fixed percentage of CMS reimbursement, others set reimbursement at a specific level for each individual code. Therefore, any comments made about relative levels of reimbursement apply only to CMS. For other third-party coverage, the only way to know what payment to expect is to check the Explanation of Benefits for each individual code.

Step 1
Identify the Patient Category

As noted in the Introduction, Step 1 is straightforward and requires only that the physician learn a few definitions and follow what is essentially a decision tree described in words. Refer frequently to the Evaluation and Management CPT Coding Guide found in Appendix A. Patient location is simply determined by where you are seeing the patient. Patient type is primarily determined by your relationship with the patient either as the treating physician or as a consultant. For most patient encounters, Step 1 will define the first four digits of the five-digit CPT code. It is the fifth digit, or level of service, that requires some effort to determine correctly and is the source of most confusion. Included in the Coding Guide is a special type of patient encounter, in which Step 1 will give you the entire five-digit code. This applies to services provided on the day of discharge of a hospitalized patient.

Step 1 is divided into two columns based on the patient location—either outpatient or inpatient. CPT describes "office or other outpatient services" as those that occur "in the physician's office or in an outpatient or other ambulatory facility (p. 1)."

Office or Other Outpatient Services

The outpatient category includes four types of patient encounters: new, established, consultation, and confirmatory consultation. The definitions for each outpatient type as determined by CPT are as follows (emphasis added):

New. "A new patient is one who has not received any professional services from the physician or another physician of the *same specialty* who belongs to the *same group practice*, within the past *three years* (p. 1)."

Established. "An established patient is one who has received professional services from the physician or another physician of the *same specialty* who belongs to the *same group practice*, within the past *three years* (p. 1)."

Consultation. "A consultation is a type of service provided by a physician whose opinion or advice regarding evaluation and/or management of a specific problem is *requested by another physician* or appropriate source (p. 13)." Consultations may be performed for either new or established patients if they meet these criteria. With regard to "appropriate source." CPT declares that consultations *cannot* be initiated by the patient or family members. An E/M service performed at the request of the patient or family members is coded as a new or established patient visit.

Confirmatory consultation. This is a consultation that is ". . . required, e.g., by a third party payor (p. 14)."

It is appropriate to make a note here about the documentation of consultations. The phrase "this patient was referred by Dr. . . ." is common medical language. Unfortunately, in the eyes of CMS, "referred" implies a transfer of care, not a request for consultation. Once a consultant becomes a treating physician, encounters are appropriately coded at the lower reimbursing new or established patient codes instead of the higher reimbursing consultation codes. A better way to document a consultation is to use CPT terminology and state "This patient is seen in consultation at the request of Dr. . . ."

Choose the correct patient type based on the definitions given above. The first four digits of the correct E/M CPT code will be as follows:

New—9920x
Established—9921x
Consultation—9924x
Confirmatory consultation—9927x

The first part of the E/M Coding Guide looks like this:

Step 1: Select appropriate patient CATEGORY and TYPE:

CATEGORY:	Outpatient	CPT
TYPE:	New	9920x
	Established	9921x
	Consultation	9924x
	Confirmatory Consult	9927x

Location Inpatient

Within the inpatient category, there are specific codes for care provided as the admitting physician and for consultation at the request of the treating physician. For hospital care as the admitting physician or in consultation, CPT further distinguishes between the first encounter with the patient and subsequent encounters. Therefore, the first four digits of the correct E/M CPT code will be as follows:

Initial hospital care (admitting physician)—9922x
Subsequent hospital care (admitting physician)—9923x

Initial in-patient consultation—9925x

Follow-up in-patient consultation—9926x

Note that CPT directs that "Only one initial consultation should be reported by a consultant per admission (p. 15)."

Hospital discharge services represent a special type of service for hospital inpatients. These codes are used to report the amount of time required to arrange for hospital discharge on the final day of the admission. Because these codes include final examination of the patient and discussions regarding the hospitalization, a separate E/M code such as 9923x should not be reported by the admitting physician on the day of discharge. Discharge day management is billed as follows:

Discharge day management less than or equal to 30 minutes—99238

Discharge day management greater than 30 minutes—99239

Step 1 of the E/M Coding Guide now looks like this:

Step 1: Select appropriate patient CATEGORY and TYPE:

CATEGORY:	Outpatient	CPT	Inpatient	CPT
TYPE:	New	9920x	Initial Hospital Care	9922x
	Established	9921x	Subsequent Hospital Care	9923x
	Consultation	9924x	Initial Inpatient Consult	9925x
	Confirmatory Consult	9927x	Follow-up Inpatient Consult	9926x
			Discharge Day Management <=30 min.	99238
			Discharge Day Management > 30 min.	99239

This completes Step 1. If you hate this entire process you can consider yourself four-fifths finished because you have four of the necessary five digits for a correct E/M CPT code. Unfortunately, determining the correct fifth digit is a little more complicated.

Reference

American Medical Association. 1997 Documentation Guidelines for Evaluation and Management Services Current Procedural Terminology CPT 2005 Standard Edition. Chicago: AMA Press, 2005.

Step 2
Use the Medical Decision-Making Table

In Step 1, we determined the patient location and patient type. For most patient encounters, this determines the first 4 digits of the 5-digit CPT code. Three components of the service determine the fifth digit: history, examination, and medical decision making. The order of these components is not random. This logical sequence of patient evaluation is taught in medical school and used in practice. First, detailed questions are asked about the chief complaint and about relevant medical problems (a history is taken). Second, a physical examination pertinent to the history is performed. After these data are gathered, a diagnosis is made and a treatment plan is formulated ("medical decision making"). The printed materials from AMA and CMS follow this well-known sequence.

This approach, however, is not the best way to understand and logically apply E/M codes. For the purposes of E/M coding according to CMS guidelines, history and examination are simply checklists of questions asked or examination components performed. It is a relatively simple matter to tally the number of items completed and determine the level of service provided. The medical decision-making component, however, has its own set of three subcomponents or elements. These three items must be ranked to determine the degree of medical decision-making "complexity" involved. The result is that the appropriate level of medical decision making is the most difficult of the three components of the fifth digit of the CPT code to determine.

While medical decision making is the most complicated component to determine according to CMS guidelines, it is actually the piece of E/M coding that should be the most intuitive. CPT describes medical decision making as "straightforward," "low complexity," "moderate complexity," and "high complexity." Without further definition of the above terms, it is probably obvious to the experienced practitioner how these terms should apply to common patient complaints for any given practice. That is, while the medical decision-making component is the most difficult to determine according to CMS guidelines, it is actually the component for which the correct level is the most obvious and intuitive based on patient presentation. Once the medical decision-making component has been determined, the history and examination can then be tailored to the appropriate level of service.

Primarily for these reasons, my method of determining correct E/M codes rearranges the traditional order of patient evaluation and makes determining the medical decision making component Step 2. History and examination are then considered sequentially in Step 3. Applying this revised order of thinking to several patient presentations that are routine in your practice is the key to understanding and accurately applying E/M codes.

To determine the degree of complexity of medical decision making, consider three elements: (1) number of diagnoses or management options, (2) amount and/or complexity of data to be reviewed, and (3) risk of complications and/or morbidity or mortality. Each of these elements will be graded on a 4-point scale. As we consider each of these elements, we will construct a grid. Once we have scored each element, the two highest ranking items will determine the degree of complexity involved.

The number of diagnoses or management options are described by AMA and CMS as "minimal," "limited," "multiple," or "extensive." The CMS Guidelines recognize that a greater number of diagnoses considered and more management options available would contribute to the complexity of medical decision making. Furthermore, management of established diagnoses is less complex than the management of new diagnoses. Comorbid conditions affect the level of medical decision making if they are directly related to the diagnosis in question (or if they increase the risk of morbidity or mortality). The first row of the Medical Decision-Making Grid looks like this:

Diagnosis and management options:	Minimal, self-limited, minor, established, stable	Limited, established, worsening	Multiple, new problem, no additional workup	Extensive, new problem, additional workup

The amount and/or complexity of data to be reviewed is also described as "minimal or none," "limited," "moderate,"or "extensive." Data review may include laboratory testing, radiographic studies, review of old medical records, and obtaining a history from someone other than the patient. Discussion with the physician who performed the test and personal review of images previously interpreted by another physician are indicators of increased complexity and should be documented. The CMS Guidelines indicate that some type of result—positive, noncontributory, an exact value, and so on—is necessary, whereas simply documenting "data reviewed" without elaboration is inadequate. With the addition of Data Review, the Medical Decision-Making Grid now looks like this:

Diagnosis and management options:	Minimal, self-limited, minor, established, stable	Limited, established, worsening	Multiple, new problem, no additional workup	Extensive, new problem, additional workup
Data review:	Minimal/ none	Limited (e.g. 1 image or lab/test)	Moderate (e.g. 1 image + lab/test)	Extensive (e.g. 2 images)

The risk of complications and/or morbidity or mortality is graded "minimal," "low," "moderate," or "high." Risk may be associated with the diagnosis itself (Presenting Problem), the diagnostic procedures required for confirmation of the diagnosis (Diagnostic Procedures Ordered), and the anticipated management options (Management Options Selected). Invasive procedures and surgery increase the amount of risk involved. Any interventions performed on an urgent basis also increase the amount of risk involved. The CMS Guidelines include a table with common clinical examples to help guide the assessment of risk (Table 2.1). The CMS Table of Risk includes examples of presenting problems, diagnostic procedures, and management options that are reflective of minimal, low, moderate, or high risk. The highest level of risk in any one of these three categories is considered the risk of complications and/or morbidity or mortality for the E/M encounter.

Table 2.1. CMS Table of Risk.

Presenting Problem(s)	One self-limited or minor problem, e.g. cold, insect bite, tinea corporis	Two or more self-limited or minor problems. One stable chronic illness, e.g. well controlled hypertension, non-insulin dependent diabetes, cataract, BPH. Acute Uncomplicated illness or injury, e.g. cystitis, allerhic rhinitis, simple sprain.	One or more chronic illnesses with mild exacerbation, progression, or side-effects of treatment. Two or more stable chronic illnesses. Undiagnosed new problem with uncertain prognosis, e.g. lump in breast. Acute illness with systemic symptoms, e.g. pyelonephritis, pneumonitis, colitis. Acute complicated injury, e.g. head injury with brief loss of conciousness.	One or more chronic illnesses with severe exacerbation, progression, or side effects of treatment. Acute or chronic illness or injuries that pose a threat to life or bodily functions, e.g. multiple trauma, acute MI, pulmonary embolus, severe respiratory distress, progressive severe rheumatoid arthritis, psychiatric illness with potential threat to self or others, peritonitis, acute renal failure.
Level of Risk	Minimal	Low	Moderate	High

(continued)

Diagnostic Procedure(s) Ordered	Laboratory testing requiring venipuncture. Chest x-rays. EKG/EEG. Urinalysis. Ultrasound, e.g. echocardiography. KOH prep.	Physiologic tests not under stress, e.g. pulmonary function tests. Non-cardiovascular imaging studies with contrast, e.g. barium enema. Superficial needle biopsies. Clinical laboratory tests requiring arterial puncture. Skin biopsies.	Physiologic tests under stress, e.g. cardiac stress test, fetal contraction stress test. Diagnostic endoscopies with no identified risk factors. Deep needle or incisional biopsy. Cardiovascular imaging studies with contrast and no identified risk factors, e.g. arteriogram, cardiac catheterization. Obtain fluid from body cavity, e.g. lumbar puncture, thoracentesis, culdocentesis.	Cardiovascular studies with contrast with identified risk factors. Cardiac electrophysiological tests. Diagnostic endoscopies with identified risk factors. Discography.
Level of Risk	Minimal	Low	Moderate	High

Management Options Selected	Rest. Gargles. Elastic bandages. Superficial dressings.	Over-the-counter drugs. Minor surgery with no identified risk factors. Physical therapy. Occupational therapy. IV fluids without additives.	Minor surgery with identified risk factors. Elective major surgery (open, percutaneous, or endoscopic) with no identified risk factors. Prescription drug management. Therapeutic nuclear medicine. IV fluids with additives. Closed treatment of fracture or dislocation without manipulation.	Elective major surgery (open, percutaneous, or endoscopic) with identified risk factors. Emergency major surgery (open, percutaneous, or endoscopic). Parenteral controlled substances. Drug therapy requiring intensive monitoring for toxicity. Decision not to resuscitate or to de-escalate care because of poor prognosis.
Level of Risk	Minimal	Low	Moderate	High

With the addition of the level of risk of complications and/or morbidity or mortality the Medical Decision Making Grid now looks like this:

Diagnosis and management options:	Minimal, self-limited, minor, established, stable	Limited, established, worsening	Multiple, new problem, no additional workup	Extensive, new problem, additional workup
Data review:	Minimal/none	Limited (e.g. 1 image or lab/test)	Moderate (e.g. 1 image + lab/test)	Extensive (e.g. 2 images)
Risk of complications/ M&M:	Minimal	Low	Moderate	High
MEDICAL DECISION MAKING	Straight-Forward	Low Complexity	Moderate Complexity	High Complexity

When using the Table of Risk, the single highest level of risk in any row determines the overall score. However, when using the Medical Decision Making Grid immediately above, each row must be scored, and it is the lower of the two highest scores that determine the overall complexity of medical decision making. Several examples follow:

Example 1. Diagnosis and management options = low complexity, data review = straight-forward complexity, risk of complications/M&M = moderate complexity. The two highest scores are low complexity and moderate complexity. The lower of these two scores is low complexity. Therefore, the overall level of medical decision making is low complexity.

Diagnosis and management options:		x (lower of two highest scores)		
Data review:	X			
Risk of complications/ M&M:			x	
MEDICAL DECISION MAKING	Straight-Forward	**Low Complexity**	Moderate Complexity	High Complexity

Example 2. Diagnosis and management options = moderate complexity, data review = moderate complexity, risk of complications/M&M = high complexity. The two highest scores are moderate complexity and high complexity. The lower of these two scores is moderate complexity. Therefore, the overall level of medical decision making is moderate complexity.

Diagnosis and management options:			x	
Data review:			x (lower of two highest scores)	
Risk of complications/ M&M:				x
MEDICAL DECISION MAKING	Straight-Forward	Low Complexity	**Moderate Complexity**	High Complexity

The correct level of medical decision making can be determined by following the steps detailed above. This is the most complicated component of E/M coding, but it is also the most closely associated to the presenting complaint. It is most easily mastered by applying this approach to the most common patient presentations in your practice. Once you have determined the level of medical decision making, the final pieces of the correct E/M code are easily assembled.

Step 3
Select the Appropriate Level for History and Examination

Step 3 requires selecting the correct level for history and physical examination. Although it might seem logical to divide these two components into two separate steps, they are both determined essentially the same way. The level of service for both history and physical are determined by counting the number of items evaluated and documented from a list determined by CMS. It is essentially the number of items that determines the correct level of service.

The patient history includes the chief complaint, history of present illness, review of systems, and past, family, and social history. (Note that with regard to E/M coding, lists of current medications are irrelevant. Allergies to medications may qualify in the "allergic/immunologic" category of the review of systems.) All E/M services require a chief complaint, defined by CMS as "a concise statement describing the symptom, problem, condition, diagnosis, physician recommended return, or other factor that is the reason for the encounter, usually stated in the patient's words." The chief complaint should be clearly stated, either separately or as the first line of the history of present illness.

The history of present illness is a chronological description of the patient's complaint, beginning with the first symptoms to the present condition. CMS recognizes the following key elements of a patient's history: location, quality, severity, duration, timing, context, modifying factors, and associated signs and symptoms. The history of present illness may be "brief" or "extended." A brief history describes one to three elements of the present illness. An extended history describes at least four elements of the present illness or at least three chronic or inactive conditions.

The review of systems is an inventory of symptoms or signs related to recognized body systems. CMS recognizes the following body systems:

1. Constitutional symptoms
2. Eyes
3. Ears, nose, mouth, throat
4. Cardiovascular
5. Respiratory
6. Gastrointestinal
7. Genitourinary
8. Musculoskeletal
9. Integumentary (skin and/or breast)
10. Neurological
11. Psychiatric
12. Endocrine
13. Hematological/lymphatic
14. Allergic/immunologic

Review of systems may be "problem pertinent," "extended," or "complete." A problem pertinent review of systems documents the system directly related to the problem detailed in the history of the present illness. An extended review of systems documents from two to nine systems, including the system pertinent to the history of the present illness. A complete review of systems documents at least ten organ systems. Pertinent positives must be recorded, however in the case of a complete system review, a notation that "all other systems are negative" is permissible.

Past medical, family, and social histories are well known to most practitioners and receive only minimal descriptions in CMS guidelines. Past history relates to "the patient's past experience with illnesses, operations, injuries, and treatments." Family history includes "a review of medical events in the patient's family, including diseases which may be hereditary or place the patient at risk." Social history involves an "age appropriate review of past and current activities." Past, family, and/or social history data gathering may be "pertinent" or "complete." A pertinent review includes one specific item relevant to the history of the present illness from any one of the three areas.

The CMS guidelines unnecessarily complicate the definition of a "complete" past, family, and/or social history review by defining it one way for some codes (two of three elements reviewed) and another way for others (three of three elements reviewed). For the sake of simplicity and to ensure compliance with the minimum guidelines in all cases, my method considers three of three elements required for a complete past, family, and social history in all cases. (The interested reader is directed to the complete CMS 1997 Documentation Guidelines for Evaluation and Management Services in Appendix D for a detailed list of codes for which two of three elements is adequate for a complete past, family, and/or social history.)

We can now determine the correct level (or type) of history taking according to CMS by tallying the number of included elements in each category. The history may be "problem focused," "expanded problem focused," "detailed," or "comprehensive." The required components for each type of history are as follows:

- A comprehensive history includes the chief complaint, four or more elements of the history of present illness ("extended"), ten or more systems reviewed ("complete"), and at least one element of past history, one element of family history, and one element of social history ("complete").

- A detailed history includes the chief complaint, four or more elements of the history of present illness ("extended"), two to nine systems reviewed ("extended"), and at least one element of past, family, and/or social history ("pertinent").

- An expanded problem focused history includes the chief complaint, one to three elements of the history of present illness ("brief"), and one related system reviewed ("problem pertinent").

- A problem focused history includes the chief complaint and one to three elements of the history of present illness ("brief").

Determination of the correct history type is shown in the table below. To qualify for a given history type, all four rows must meet or exceed the given requirements.

History of Present Illness	Chief Complaint			
	1–3 elements	1–3 elements	4 or more elements	4 or more elements
Review of Systems	None required	1 related	2–9 systems	10 or more systems
Past, Family, and/or Social History	None required	None required	1 or more element(s) (1/3)	1 of each element (3/3)
Type of History	Problem Focused	Expanded Problem Focused	Detailed	Comprehensive

As summarized in the Coding Guide (Appendix A) the type of history is as follows:

HISTORY:

Comprehensive	CC, HPI >=4 elements, ROS >=10 systems, PFSH 3/3
Detailed	CC, HPI >=4 elements, ROS 2–9 systems, PFSH 1/3
Expanded Problem Focused	CC, HPI 1–3 elements, ROS 1 related
Problem Focused	CC, HPI 1–3 elements

CMS applies nomenclature similar to that used for the type of history to the level (or type) of examination. The physical examination may be problem focused, expanded problem focused, detailed, or comprehensive. For the purposes of E/M coding CMS recognizes the following distinct categories of examination:

1. General multi-system
2. Cardiovascular
3. Ears, Nose, Mouth, and Throat
4. Eyes
5. Genitourinary (Female)
6. Genitourinary (Male)
7. Hematologic/Lymphatic/Immunologic
8. Musculoskelatal
9. Neurological
10. Psychiatric
11. Respiratory
12. Skin

The content of each examination, general multi-system or single organ system, is described by CMS in the 1997 Guidelines in table form. For purposes of illustration, the general multi-system examination and the neurological examination will be discussed in detail. The complete examination guidelines are shown in Appendix D.

The general multi-system examination recognizes 14 systems or body areas. Each system or body area has two or more elements of examination identified as bullet points. The first two systems or body areas of the general mutisystem examination are shown below:

System/Body Area	Elements of Examination
Constitutional	• Measurement of any three of the following seven vital signs: (1) sitting or standing blood pressure, (2) supine blood pressure, (3) pulse rate and regularity, (4) respiration, (5) temperature, (6) height, (7) weight (May be measured and recorded by ancillary staff). • General appearance of patient (e.g. development, nutrition, body habitus, deformities, attention to grooming).
Eyes	• Inspection of conjunctivae and lids. • Examination of pupils and irises (e.g. reaction to light and accommodation, size, and symmetry). • Ophthalmologic examination of optic discs (e.g. size, C/D ratio, appearance) and posterior segments (e.g. vessel changes, exudates, hemorrhages).

Each bullet point identifies a single element of the examination. For some elements, such as vital signs, a certain number of components must be documented. Elements with multiple components but no specific numeric requirement (e.g. examination of pupils and irises) require documentation of at least one component.

The complete general multi-system examination is as follows:

System/Body Area	Elements of Examination
Constitutional	• Measurement of any three of the following seven vital signs: (1) sitting or standing blood pressure, (2) supine blood pressure, (3) pulse rate and regularity, (4) respiration, (5) temperature, (6) height, (7) weight (May be measured and recorded by ancillary staff). • General appearance of patient (e.g. development, nutrition, body habitus, deformities, attention to grooming).
Eyes	• Inspection of conjunctivae and lids. • Examination of pupils and irises (e.g. reaction to light and accommodation, size, and symmetry). • Ophthalmologic examination of optic discs (e.g. size, C/D ratio, appearance) and posterior segments (e.g. vessel changes, exudates, hemorrhages).
Ears, Nose, Mouth, and Throat	• External inspection of ears and nose (e.g. overall appearance, scars, lesions, masses) • Otoscopic examination of external auditory canals and tympanic membranes • Assesment of hearing (e.g. whispered voice, finger rub, tuning fork)

(continued)

	• Inspection of nasal mucosa, septum, and turbinates • Inspection of lips, teeth, and gums • Examination of oropharynx: oral mucosa, salivary glands, hard and soft palates, tongue, tonsils, and posterior pharynx
Neck	• Examination of neck (e.g. masses, overall appearance, symmetry, tracheal position, crepitus) • Examination of thyroid (e.g. enlargement, tenderness, mass)
Respiratory	• Assessment of respiratory effort (e.g. intercostals retractions, use of accessory muscles, diaphragmatic movement) • Percussion of chest (e.g. dullness, flatness, hyperresonance) • Palpation of chest (e.g. tactile fremitus) • Auscultation of lungs (e.g. breath sounds, adventitious sounds, rubs)
Cardiovascular	• Palpation of heart (e.g. location, size, thrills) • Auscultation of heart with notation of abnormal sounds and murmurs Examination of: • carotid arteries (e.g. pulse amplitude, bruits) • abdominal aorta (e.g. size, bruits) • femoral arteries (e.g. pulse amplitude, bruits) • pedal pulses (e.g. pulse amplitude) • extremities for edema and/or varicosities
Chest (Breasts)	• Inspection of breasts (e.g. symmetry, nipple discharge) • Palpation of breasts and axillae (e.g. masses or lumps, tenderness)

Gastrointestinal (Abdomen)	• Examination of abdomen with notation of presence of masses or tenderness • Examination of liver and spleen • Examination for presence or absence of hernia • Examination (when indicated) of anus, perineum and rectum, including sphincter tone, presence of hemorrhoids, rectal masses • Obtain stool sample for occult blood test when indicated
Genitourinary	**Male:** • Examination of scrotal contents (e.g. hydrocele, spermatocele, tenderness of cord, testicular mass) • Examination of the penis • Digital rectal examination of prostate gland (e.g. size, symmetry, nodularity, tenderness) **Female:** Pelvic examination (with or without specimen collection for smears and cultures), including: • Examination of external genitalia (e.g. general appearance, hair distribution, lesions) and vagina (e.g. general appearance, estrogen effect, discharge, lesions, pelvic support, cystocele, rectocele) • Examination of urethra (e.g. masses, tenderness, scarring) • Examination of bladder (e.g. fullness, masses, tenderness) • Cervix (e.g. general appearance, lesions, discharge) • Uterus (e.g. size, contour, position, mobility, tenderness, consistency, descent or support) • Adnexa/parametria (e.g. masses, tenderness, organomegaly, nodularity)

(continued)

Lymphatic	Palpation of lymph nodes in two or more areas: • Neck • Axillae • Groin • Other
Musculoskeletal	• Examination of gait and station • Inspection and/or palpation of digits and nails (e.g. clubbing, cyanosis, inflammatory conditions, petechiae, ischemia, infections, nodes) Examination of joints, bones, and muscles of one or more of the following six areas: (1) head and neck; (2) spine, ribs and pelvis; (3) right upper extremity; (4) left upper extremity; (5) right lower extremity; (6) left lower extremity. The examination of a given area includes: • Inspection and/or palpation with notation of presence of any misalignment, asymmetry, crepitation, defects, tenderness, masses, effusions • Assessment of range of motion with notation of any pain, crepitation, or contracture • Assessment of stability with notation of any dislocation (luxation), subluxation, or laxity • Assessment of muscle strength and tone (e.g. flaccid, cog wheel, spastic) with notation of any atrophy or abnormal movements

Skin	• Inspection of skin and subcutaneous tissue (e.g. rashes, lesions, ulcers) • Palpation of skin and subcutaneous tissue (e.g. induration, subcutaneous nodules, tightening)
Neurologic	• Test cranial nerves with notation of any deficits • Examination of deep tendon reflexes with notation of pathological reflexes (e.g. Babinski) • Examination of sensation (e.g. by touch, pin, vibration, proprioception)
Psychiatric	• Description of patient's judgement and insight Brief assessment of mental status including: • orientation to time, place, and person • recent and remote memory • mood and affect (e.g. depression, anxiety, agitation)

The CMS guidelines contain a set of criteria used for determining the type of examination performed when using the general multi-system examination. Unfortunately, here again CMS seems to add unnecessary complications by proscribing slightly different criteria for exam type if the practitioner is using a single organ system examination. It is easier to understand these differences if we first review a single organ system examination, noting the differences in structure between it and the general exam. After doing that, it is relatively simple to construct a set of guidelines that meet CMS requirements regardless of the type of examination that is being used.

Shown below are the first six systems/body areas of the neurological examination, "Constitutional," "Head and Face," "Eyes," and so on.

System/Body Area	Elements of Examination
Constitutional	• Measurement of any three of the following seven vital signs: (1) sitting or standing blood pressure, (2) supine blood pressure, (3) pulse rate and regularity, (4) respiration, (5) temperature, (6) height, (7) weight (may be measured and recorded by ancillary staff). • General appearance of patient (e.g. development, nutrition, body habitus, deformities, attention to grooming).
Head and Face	
Eyes	• Ophthalmologic examination of optic discs (e.g. size, C/D ratio, appearance) and posterior segments (e.g. vessel changes, exudates, hemorrhages).
Ears, Nose, Mouth and Throat	
Neck	
Respiratory	
Cardiovascular	• Examination of carotid arteries (e.g. pulse, amplitude, bruits) • Auscultation of heart with notation of normal sounds and murmurs • Examination of peripheral vascular system by observation (e.g. swelling, varicosities) and palpation (e.g. pulses, temperature, edema, tenderness)

Comparing these first six systems/body areas to the general multi-system examination a number of differences become apparent:

1. Some of the systems/body areas (Constitutional and Eyes in this example) have a shaded border.

2. While the elements of the Constitutional system are identical with those of the general multi-system examination, the "Eyes" section eliminates some of the elements from the general examination. The "Cardiovascular" section lumps the examination of the peripheral vascular system into one element, whereas in the general examination it was divided into five individual elements.

3. A body area absent in the general multi-system examination shows up in the single organ system ("Head and Face")

4. Some of the systems/body areas (e.g. Head and Face) have no elements in them. The importance of these differences will become apparent when we generate a set of rules that both conform to CMS guidelines but are applicable regardless of the examination template used.

Shown below is the complete Neurological Examination.

System/Body Area	Elements of Examination
Constitutional	• Measurement of any three of the following seven vital signs: (1) sitting or standing blood pressure, (2) supine blood pressure, (3) pulse rate and regularity, (4) respiration, (5) temperature, (6) height, (7) weight (May be measured and recorded by ancillary staff). • General appearance of patient (e.g. development, nutrition, body habitus, deformities, attention to grooming).

Head and Face	
Eyes	• Ophthalmologic examination of optic discs (e.g. size, C/D ratio, appearance) and posterior segments (e.g. vessel changes, exudates, hemorrhages).
Ears, Nose, Mouth, and Throat	
Neck	
Respiratory	
Cardiovascular	• Examination of carotid arteries (e.g. pulse amplitude, bruits) • Auscultation of heart with notation of abnormal sounds and murmurs • Examination of peripheral vascular system by observation (e.g. swelling, varicosities) and palpation (e.g. pulses, temperature, edema, tenderness)
Chest (Breasts)	
Gastrointestinal (Abdomen)	
Genitourinary	
Lymphatic	
Musculoskelatal	• Examination of gait and station Assesment of motor function including: • Muscle strength in upper and lower extremities • Muscle tone in upper and lower extremities (e.g. flaccid, cog wheel, spastic) with notation of any atrophy or abnormal movements (e.g. fasciculation, tardive dyskinesia)
Extremities	[See musculoskeletal]

Skin	
Neurologic	Evaluation of higher integrative function including: • Orientation to time, place, and person • Recent and remote memory • Attention span and concentration • Language (e.g. naming objects, repeating phrases, spontaneous speech) Test the following cranial nerves: • 2nd cranial nerve (e.g. visual acuity, visual fields, fundi) • 3rd, 4th, and 6th cranial nerves (e.g. pupils, eye movements) • 5th cranial nerve (e.g. facial sensation, corneal reflex) • 7th cranial nerve (e.g. facial symmetry, strength) • 8th cranial nerve (e.g. hearing with tuning fork, whispered voice and finger rub) • 9th cranial nerve (e.g. spontaneous or reflex palate movement) • 11th cranial nerve (e.g. shoulder shrug strength) • 12th cranial nerve (e.g. tongue protrusion) • Examination of sensation (e.g. by touch, pin, vibration, proprioception) • Examination of deep tendon reflexes in upper and lower extremities with notation of pathological reflexes (e.g. Babinski) • Test coordination (e.g. finger to nose, heel/knee/shin, rapid alternating movements in the upper and lower extremities, evaluation of fine motor coordination in young children)
Psychiatric	

One more difference between the general multi-system examination and the single organ system examination is now apparent. The organ system, for which the specialty exam is named ("neurological" in this example), is significantly expanded. The complete single organ system examinations for the following systems are shown in Appendix D: eye; ear, nose, and throat; respiratory; cardiovascular; genitourinary; hematologic/lymphatic/immunologic; musculoskeletal; skin; neurological; and psychiatric.

Now we can consider the requirements for each type of examination and generate a set of criteria that meet CMS guidelines whether one is performing a general mutisystem or single organ system examination.

Problem Focused Examination

For either the general multi-system or the single organ system examination, CMS requires documentation of one to five elements identified by a bullet (•).

Expanded Problem Focused Examination

For either the general multi-system or the single organ system examination, CMS requires documentation of at least six elements identified by a bullet (•).

Detailed Examination

For the general multi-system examination, CMS requires ". . . at least six organ systems or body areas. For each system/area selected performance and documentation of at least two elements identified by a bullet (•) is expected. Alternatively, a detailed examination may include performance and documentation of at least twelve elements identified by a bullet (•) in two or more organ systems or body areas."

For the single organ system examination, CMS requires ". . . performance and documentation of at least twelve elements identified by a bullet (•), whether in a box with a shaded or unshaded border. An exception is made for the Eye and Psychiatric single organ system examinations, each of which requires at least nine elements identified by a bullet (•) whether in a box with a shaded or unshaded border for a detailed examination.

Using the "alternatively" acceptable guidelines for the general multi-system examination, the CMS requirements for a detailed examination can be met for either a general multi-system or single organ system examination by documenting at least twelve elements identified by a bullet.

Comprehensive Examination

For the general multi-system examination, CMS requires ". . . at least nine organ systems or body areas. For each system/area selected, all elements of the examination identified by a bullet (•) should be performed, unless specific directions limit the content of the examination. For each area/system, documentation of at least two elements identified by a bullet is expected." Notice that the CMS requirements dictate performance of every component of the examination identified by a bullet in nine areas but only require documentation of two of those elements. Presumably this means that if the gastrointestinal system is included in the general examination all five elements must be performed but only two must be documented to meet CMS guidelines.

For the single organ system examination, CMS requires ". . . performance of all elements identified by a bullet (•), whether in a shaded or unshaded box. Documentation of every element in each box with a shaded border and at least one element in each box with an unshaded border is expected.

Since my method and the Code Guide shown in Appendix A are concerned solely with meeting documentation guidelines, and not with performance standards, the summary statements for the Comprehensive Examination are as follows:

General multi-system: at least two elements from each of nine systems/areas.

Single organ system: every element in shaded box and at least one element in unshaded box.

As summarized in the Coding Guide (Appendix A), the examination type is as follows:

EXAMINATION:

Comprehensive	General multi-system: at least two elements from each of nine systems/areas. Single organ system: every element in shaded box and at least one element in unshaded box.
Detailed	At least 12 elements identified by a bullet*.
Expanded Problem Focused	At least 6 elements identified by a bullet.
Problem Focused	5 elements identified by a bullet.

*Eye and psychiatric examinations require at least nine elements.

Using the information in this chapter, we now know the type of history and examination. Combined with the patient location and type from Step 1 and the level of medical decision making from Step 2, we are ready to determine the correct CPT code for the level of E/M service provided.

Step 4
Identify the Correct CPT Code and Modifier

Using the data collected in the previous three steps, the correct E/M CPT code can be determined. In Step 1, the patient location and type were identified. These two characteristics gave us the first four digits of the correct code. In Step 2, the level of medical decision making involved in the encounter was determined. Medical decision making can be straightforward (SF), low complexity (LC), moderate complexity (MC), or high complexity (HC). In Step 3, the levels of history and examination were determined. Both may be problem focused (PF), expanded problem focused (EPF), detailed (DET), or comprehensive (COMP).

For each patient location and type there are three to five levels of service that may be provided. Each level of service is defined by the medical decision making, history, and examination involved. CPT requires that each of these three categories meet or exceed a certain threshold to qualify for a given E/M code. For example, to qualify for a level "3" code service provided to a new patient seen in the office (9920x) would require low complexity medical decision making, a detailed history, and a detailed examination. In table form, this is shown as:

CPI	MDM	Hx	Exam
99203	LC	Det	Det

The five levels of service that may be provided to a new patient seen in the office or other outpatient setting are shown as:

CPT	MDM	Hx	Exam
99201	SF	PF	PF
99202	SF	EPF	EPF
99203	LC	Det	Det
99204	MC	Comp	Comp
99205	HC	Comp	Comp

Remember that in determining the correct E/M code, the level of service must meet or exceed requirements in all three categories. For example, a comprehensive history, comprehensive examination, and straightforward medical decision making qualifies only for a level "2" code, whereas the same history and examination with moderate complexity medical decision making qualifies for a level 4 code.

Including both of the patient locations and all of the patient types described in Step 1, the E/M CPT code table looks like this:

CPT	MDM	Hx	Exam	CPT	MDM	Hx	Exam	CPT	MDM	Hx	Exam
99201	SF	PF	PF	99221	Low	Det	Det	99241	SF	PF	PF
99202	SF	EPF	EPF	99222	MC	Comp	Comp	99242	SF	EPF	EPF
99203	LC	Det	Det	99223	HC	Comp	Comp	99243	LC	Det	Det
99204	MC	Comp	Comp					99244	MC	Comp	Comp
99205	HC	Comp	Comp	99231	Low	PF	PF	99245	HC	Comp	Comp
99211	No physician required			99232	MC	EPF	EPF	99251	SF	PF	PF
99212	SF	PF	PF	99233	HC	Det	Det	99252	SF	EPF	EPF
99213	LC	EPF	EPF					99253	LC	Det	Det
99214	MC	Det	Det					99254	MC	Comp	Comp
99215	HC	Comp	Comp					99255	HC	Comp	Comp

As noted in the introduction, CMS publishes RVU information and conversion factors for all CPT codes. Using this information, an estimate of expected reimbursement from CMS for various services can be calculated. This estimate does not take into account geographic adjustments or adjustments made for practicing in an underserved location. As an example, consider two patient visits. Patient A is an established patient seen in the office for follow up of a chronic, stable problem. With a problem-focused history, problem-focused examination, and straightforward medical decision making, this patient qualifies for a level 2 established patient visit—99212. If CMS assigns 1.01 RVU to 99212 and reimburses $38.50 per RVU, a practitioner can expect to receive $38.89 in compensation for the care provided to patient A. Patient B is a patient seen in the hospital at the request of another physician for a new problem. A comprehensive history and a comprehensive examination were performed. Medical decision making was of moderate complexity, and this patient qualifies for a level 4 inpatient consultation—99254. If CMS assigns 3.76 RVU the practitioner can expect to receive $144.76 for the services provided.

A final component of correct coding is the use of modifiers. From the provider's perspective, modifiers have two useful purposes. They may either justify the submission of charges for a service that might otherwise not be indicated, or they may increase the value of a service in an encounter that is, for some reason, not routine. Some modifiers are specific to procedure codes, e.g. "-62 Two Surgeons." Following is a list of codes that are more applicable to E/M services. The definitions are directly from the AMA:

-21 Prolonged Evaluation and Management Services: When the face-to-face or floor/unit service(s) provided is prolonged or otherwise greater than that usually required for the highest level of evaluation and management service within a given category, it may be identified by adding modifier 21 to the evaluation and management code number. A report may also be appropriate.

-24 Unrelated Evaluation and Management Service by the Same Physician During a Postoperative Period: (Many surgical procedures include a postoperative global period within which reimbursement for all routine postoperative care is included in the surgical fee.) The physician may need to indicate that an evaluation and management service was performed during a postoperative period for a reason(s) unrelated to the original procedure. This circumstance may be reported by adding modifier 24 to the appropriate level of E/M service.

-25 Significant, Separately Identifiable Evaluation and Management Service by the Same Physician on the Same Day of the Procedure or other Service: The physician may need to indicate that on the day a procedure or service identified by a CPT code was performed, the patient's condition required a significant, separately identifiable E/M service above and beyond the other service provided or beyond the usual preoperative and postoperative care associated with the procedure performed. A significant, separately identifiable E/M service is defined or substantiated by documentation that satisfies the relevant criteria for the respective E/M services to be reported. The E/M service may be prompted by the symptom or condition for which the procedure and/or service was provided. As such, different diagnoses are not required for reporting of the E/M services on the same date. This circumstance may be reported by adding modifier 25 to the appropriate level of E/M service. This modifier is not used to report an E/M service that resulted in a decision to perform surgery. See modifier 57.

-32 Mandated Services: Services related to mandated consultation and/or related services (e.g. PRO, third party payer,
governmental, legislative, or regulatory requirement) may
be identified by adding the modifier 32 to the basic
procedure.

-57 Decision for Surgery: An evaluation and management
service that resulted in the initial decision to perform
surgery may be identified by adding modifier 57 to the
appropriate level of E/M service.

The modifiers shown above should be added to the E/M code
when appropriate and supported by documentation. For example,
a level 4 new patient visit that resulted in a decision to proceed
with surgery would be coded "99204-57". A level 3 evaluation of
low back pain in a patient treated surgically six weeks ago (within
the 90 day postoperative global period) for cervical disk hernia-
tion would be coded "99213-24."

Appendices

Appendix A
E/M Coding Guide*

Christopher L. Taylor, MD

Step 1: Select appropriate patient LOCATION and TYPE:

LOCATION:	Outpatient	CPT	Inpatient	CPT
TYPE:	New	9920x	Initial Hospital Care	9922x
	Established	9921x	Subsequent Hospital Care	9923x
	Consultation	9924x	Initial Inpatient Consult	9925x
	Confirmatory Consult	9927x	Follow-up Inpatient Consult	9926x
			Discharge Day Management <= 30 min.	99238
			Discharge Day Management > 30 min.	99239

Step 2: Determine the level of MEDICAL DECISION MAKING that meets or exceeds two of the three components in the following table:

51

Table A.1. Medical decision making.

Diagnosis and management options:	Self-limited, minor, established, stable	Established, worsening	New problem, no additional workup	New problem, additional workup
Risk of complications/ M&M:	Minimal	Low	Moderate	High
Data review:	Minimal/ none	1 Image	1 Image + lab/test	2 Images
MEDICAL DECISION MAKING	Straight-Forward	Low Complexity	Moderate Complexity	High Complexity

Step 3: Determine the level of the HISTORY and the EXAMINATION

HISTORY:

Comprehensive   CC, HPI >= 4 elements, ROS >= 10 systems, PFSH 3/3

Detailed   CC, HPI >= 4 elements, ROS 2–9 systems, PFSH 1/3

Expanded **P**roblem Focused   CC, HPI 1–3 elements, ROS 1 related

Problem **F**ocused   CC, HPI 1–3 elements

EXAMINATION:

Comprehensive   All elements identified by a bullet; every element with a bold underline and at least one element with a un-bolded underline.

Detailed   At least 12 elements identified by a bullet.

Expanded **P**roblem Focused   At least 6 elements identified by a bullet.

Problem **F**ocused   5 elements identified by a bullet.

Step 4: Determine the appropriate CPT code and MODIFIER from the following table:

Table A.2. CPT codes.

CPT	MDM	Hx	Exam	CPT	MDM	Hx	Exam	CPT	MDM	Hx	Exam
99201	SF	PF	PF	99231	Low	PF	PF	99261	Low	PF	PF
99202	SF	EPF	EPF	99232	MC	EPF	EPF	99262	MC	EPF	EPF
99203	LC	Det	Det	99233	HC	Det	Det	99263	HC	Det	Det
99204	MC	Comp	Comp	99241	SF	PF	PF	99271	SF	PF	PF
99205	HC	Comp	Comp	99242	SF	EPF	EPF	99272	SF	EPF	EPF
99211	No physician required			99243	LC	Det	Det	99273	LC	Det	Det
99212	SF	PF	PF	99244	MC	Comp	Comp	99274	MC	Comp	Comp
99213	LC	EPF	EPF	99245	HC	Comp	Comp	99275	HC	Comp	Comp
99214	MC	Det	Det	99251	SF	PF	PF	99281	SF	PF	PF
99215	HC	Comp	Comp	99252	SF	EPF	EPF	99282	LC	EPF	EPF
99221	Low	Det	Det	99253	LC	Det	Det	99283	MC	EPF	EPF
99222	MC	Comp	Comp	99254	MC	Comp	Comp	99284	MC	Det	Det
99223	HC	Comp	Comp	99255	HC	Comp	Comp	99285	HC	Comp	Comp

Modifiers:
*CPT (Current Procedural Terminology) codes are copyright of American Medical Association.

Appendix B
New Patient Consultation
Template: Neurosurgical Practice

Christopher L. Taylor, MD

Authors note: This is a complete evaluation for new patients seen in my neurosurgical practice. The history section is comprehensive including an identifying statement, at least four elements of the history of present illness, eleven systems reviewed, past, family, and social history. The examination includes all of the required elements for a comprehensive neurological examination. If supported by the level of medical decision making, this E/M template will meet the requirements for a new patient visit or consultation up to a level 5.

Dictation Template

> *Note to transcriptionist:* Items in (parenthesis) are prompts for the doctor and should be left blank if not dictated. Items that are <u>underlined</u> should be changed *if noted in the dictation.*

Chief complaint: This is a (age) year-old (right-handed/left-handed) (man/woman) (seen at the request of Dr. name) with a chief complaint of (chief complaint).

History of present illness: (History of present illness, including at least four of the following: Location, Duration, Quality, Timing, Severity, Modifying Factors, Context, Associated Symptoms and Signs).

Review of systems (All items denied except those specifically mentioned in dictation):

Constitutional: fever: <u>denies</u>, weight loss: <u>denies</u>

Eyes: vision loss: <u>denies</u>, double vision: <u>denies</u>

Ears, nose, mouth, throat: hearing loss: <u>denies</u>, tinnitus: <u>denies</u>, nasal drainage: <u>denies</u> hoarseness: <u>denies</u>, difficulty swallowing: <u>denies</u>

Cardiovascular: chest pain: <u>denies</u>, chest pain with exertion: <u>denies</u>

Respiratory: shortness of breath: <u>denies</u>, cough: <u>denies</u>

Gastrointestinal: blood in stool: <u>denies</u>, constipation: <u>denies</u>

Genitourinary: incontinence: <u>denies</u>, sexual dysfunction: <u>denies</u>

Musculoskeletal: muscle pain: <u>denies</u>, joint pain: <u>denies</u>

Neurological: headache: <u>denies</u>, numbness: <u>denies</u>, tingling: <u>denies</u>, tremor: <u>denies</u>

Endocrine: heat/cold intolerance: <u>denies</u>, change in ring/shoe size: <u>denies</u>

Hematologic/Lymphatic: easy bleeding: <u>denies</u>, easy bruising: <u>denies</u>

Past history: (Dictate past medical and past surgical history.)

Family history: (Dictate health status of immediate family.)

Social history: (Dictate marital status, current employment, alcohol, tobacco, recreational drug use.)

Medications: (Dictate pertinent medications.)

Drug allergies: (Dictate known allergies.)

Neurological Examination

Constitutional
- Vital signs: (3 of the following: 1- blood pressure 2- pulse rate and regularity 3- respiration 4- temperature 5- height 6- weight)
- General appearance: <u>well developed, well nourished, age appropriate</u>

Eyes
- Ophthalmoscopic exam of optic discs and posterior segments (fundi): <u>normal size, no papilledema</u>

Cardiovascular
- Carotid arteries: pulse amplitude <u>not examined</u>, bruits <u>not examined</u>
- Peripheral vascular system: <u>no swelling or varicosities, no edema, warm, non-tender</u>
  Right posterior tibial pulse: <u>not examined</u>, Right dorsalis pedis pulse: <u>not examined</u>
  Left posterior tibial pulse: <u>not examined</u>, Left dorsalis pedis pulse: <u>not examined</u>

Musculoskeletal
- Gait and station: <u>normal</u>
- Muscle strength:

  Right delt. <u>5/5</u>; biceps <u>5/5</u>; triceps <u>5/5</u>; flex. pol. <u>5/5</u>; oppon. pol. <u>5/5</u>; intrinsics <u>5/5</u>
  Left delt. <u>5/5</u>; biceps <u>5/5</u>; triceps <u>5/5</u>; flex. pol. <u>5/5</u>; oppon. pol. <u>5/5</u>; intrinsics <u>5/5</u>
  Right thigh add. <u>5/5</u>; quad. <u>5/5</u>; ant. tib. <u>5/5</u>; EHL <u>5/5</u>; gastroc./evertors <u>5/5</u>
  Left thigh add. <u>5/5</u>; quad. <u>5/5</u>; ant. tib. <u>5/5</u>; EHL <u>5/5</u>; gastroc./evertors <u>5/5</u>

- Muscle tone: normal bulk and tone, no atrophy or abnormal movements

Neurological

Evaluation of higher integrative functions:
- Orientation to time, place, and person: intact
- Recent and remote memory: intact
- Attention span and concentration: intact
- Language: normal naming, repetition, and spontaneous speech
- Fund of knowledge for current events, past history, and vocabulary: normal

Cranial nerves:
- 2nd CN: visual acuity was not tested
  Visual fields: intact to confrontation
  Fundus examination recorded under "ophthalmoscopic exam" above.
- 3rd, 4th, & 6th CN: pupils equal and reactive to light, extraocular movements intact
- 5th CN: facial sensation intact, masseter muscle normal (note corneal reflex)
- 7th CN: face symmetric
- 8th CN: hearing intact bilateral to finger rub
- 9th and 10th CN: uvula and palate elevate normally in the midline (note gag reflex)
- 11th CN: shoulder shrug normal bilateral
- 12th CN: tongue protrudes in the midline

Other neurological:
- Sensation: light touch intact througout (note decrease, radicular distribution)
  Pin prick: intact througout (note decrease, radicular distribution, sensory level)

(Note straight leg raise, vibration, proprioception, Tinel
    sign, Phalen test)
- Deep tendon reflexes: right biceps <u>2+</u>, right triceps <u>2+</u>;
    left biceps <u>2+</u>, left triceps <u>2+;</u> right knee <u>2+</u>, right ankle
    <u>2+;</u> left knee <u>2+</u>, left ankle <u>2+;</u> Babinski sign: <u>absent
    bilateral</u>
    (Note Hoffman sign, ankle clonus)
- Coordination: finger to nose <u>intact bilateral</u>, heel to
    shin <u>intact bilateral</u> (Note rapid alternating movements,
    Romberg sign).

Medical Decision Making
(Note type and date of images independently reviewed, image
reports reviewed, need to obtain history from someone other than
the patient, clinical lab tests reviewed, other tests or studies
reviewed, discussion of tests with performing MD.)

Diagnosis: (ICD-9 code, differential diagnosis)
Plan for care: (Note risk of complications and/or morbidity
    and mortality, risks and benefits of different management
    options, recommendation.)

Appendix C
New Patient Consultation
Template: Low Back Pain

Christopher L. Taylor, MD

Authors note: This is a limited evaluation for new patients seen in my neurosurgical practice with uncomplicated low back pain. The history section includes an identifying statement, a history of present illness, three systems reviewed, and social history. The examination includes twelve elements from more than two systems therefore qualifying for a detailed general multisystem examination. If supported by the level of medical decision making, this E/M template will meet the requirements for a new patient visit or consultation up to a level 3.

Dictation Template

Note to transcriptionist: Items in (parenthesis) are prompts for the doctor and should be left blank if not dictated. Items that are <u>underlined</u> should be changed if noted in the dictation.

(Ask transcriptionist to use **Low Back** template.)

> **Chief complaint:** This is a (age) year-old (man/woman) (seen at the request of Dr. name) with a chief complaint of (chief complaint).
>
> **History of present illness:** (History of present illness including at least four of the following: Location, Duration, Quality, Timing, Severity, Modifying Factors, Context, Associated Symptoms and Signs.) (Dictate treatment prior to evaluation including medications, physical therapy, etc.)
>
> **Review of systems** (All items denied except those specifically mentioned in dictation):
>
> *Genitourinary:* incontinence: denies, sexual dysfunction: denies
>
> *Musculoskeletal:* muscle pain: denies, joint pain: denies
>
> *Neurological:* headache: denies, numbness: denies, tingling: denies, tremor: denies
>
> **Social history:** (Dictate current employment and tobacco use.)
>
> **Medications:** (Dictate pertinent medications.)
>
> **Drug allergies:** (Dictate known allergies.)

Physical Examination

Constitutional
- Vital signs: (1- pulse rate 2- height 3- weight)
- General appearance: well developed, well nourished, age-appropriate

Cardiovascular
- Peripheral vascular system: no swelling or varicosities, no edema, warm, non-tender

Right posterior tibial pulse: <u>2+</u>, Right dorsalis pedis pulse: <u>2+</u>

Left posterior tibial pulse: <u>2+</u>, Left dorsalis pedis pulse: <u>2+</u>

Musculoskeletal

- Gait and station: <u>normal, non-tender to palpation of the thoracic and lumbar spine, no pain with lateral bending</u>
- Muscle strength:

    Right thigh add. <u>5/5</u>; quad. <u>5/5</u>; ant. tib. <u>5/5</u>; EHL <u>5/5</u>; gastroc./evertors <u>5/5</u>

    Left thigh add. <u>5/5</u>; quad. <u>5/5</u>; ant. tib. <u>5/5</u>; EHL <u>5/5</u>; gastroc./evertors <u>5/5</u>

- Muscle tone: <u>normal bulk and tone, no atrophy or abnormal movements</u>

Neurological

Evaluation of higher integrative functions:
- Orientation to time, place, and person: <u>intact</u>
- Recent and remote memory: <u>intact</u>
- Attention span and concentration: <u>intact</u>
- Language: <u>normal naming, repetition, and spontaneous speech</u>
- Fund of knowledge for current events, past history, and vocabulary: <u>normal</u>

Other neurological:
- Sensation: light touch <u>intact</u> (note decrease, radicular distribution)

    Pin prick: <u>intact</u> (note decrease, radicular distribution, sensory level)

    <u>Straight leg raise negative bilateral</u>

- Deep tendon reflexes: right knee <u>2+</u>, right ankle <u>2+;</u> left knee <u>2+</u>, left ankle <u>2+;</u> Babinski sign <u>absent bilateral, no ankle clonus</u>

Medical Decision Making

(Note type and date of images independently reviewed, image reports reviewed, need to obtain history from someone other than the patient, clinical lab tests reviewed, other tests or studies reviewed, discussion of tests with performing MD.)

Diagnosis: (ICD-9 code, differential diagnosis)

Plan for care: (Note risk of complications and/or morbidity and mortality, risks and benefits of different management options, medications given, recommendation.)

Appendix D
1997 Documentation Guidelines for Evaluation and Management Services*

*www.cms.hhs.gov/MLNProducts/Downloads/MASTER1.pdf
(Accessed June 29, 2006)

REFERENCE II

1997 DOCUMENTATION GUIDELINES
FOR EVALUATION & MANAGEMENT SERVICES

TABLE OF CONTENTS

Introduction 2

What Is Documentation and Why Is it Important? 2

What Do Payers Want and Why? 2

General Principles of Medical Record Documentation 3

Documentation of E/M Services...4

Documentation of History 5

Chief Complaint (CC) 6

History of Present Illness (HPI) 7

Review of Systems (ROS) 8

Past, Family and/or Social History (PFSH) 9

Documentation of Examination 10

General Multi-System Examinations 11

Single Organ System Examinations 12

Content and Documentation Requirements 13

General Multi-System Examination 13
    Cardiovascular Examination 18
    Ear, Nose and Throat Examination 20
    Eye Examination 23
    Genitourinary Examination 26
    Hematologic/Lymphatic/Immunologic Examination 29
    Musculoskeletal Examination 32
    Neurological Examination 35

Psychiatric Examination 38
Respiratory Examination 39
Skin Examination 42

Documentation of the Complexity of Medical Decision Making 43

Number of Diagnoses or Management Options 44

Amount and/or Complexity of Data to Be Reviewed 45

Risk of Significant Complications, Morbidity, and/or Mortality 46

Table of Risk 47

Documentation of an Encounter Dominated by Counseling or Coordination
of Care 48

I. INTRODUCTION

WHAT IS DOCUMENTATION AND WHY IS IT IMPORTANT?

Medical record documentation is required to record pertinent facts, findings, and observations about an individual's health history including past and present illnesses, examinations, tests, treatments, and outcomes. The medical record chronologically documents the care of the patient and is an important element contributing to high quality care. The medical record facilitates:

- the ability of the physician and other healthcare professionals to evaluate and plan the patient's immediate treatment, and to monitor his/her healthcare over time.

- communication and continuity of care among physicians and other healthcare professionals involved in the patient's care;

- accurate and timely claims review and payment;

- appropriate utilization review and quality of care evaluations; and

- collection of data that may be useful for research and education.

An appropriately documented medical record can reduce many of the hassles associated with claims processing and may serve as a legal document to verify the care provided, if necessary.

WHAT DO PAYERS WANT AND WHY?

Because payers have a contractual obligation to enrollees, they may require reasonable documentation that services are consistent with the insurance coverage provided. They may request information to validate:

- the site of service;

- the medical necessity and appropriateness of the diagnostic and/or therapeutic services provided; and/or

- that services provided have been accurately reported.

II. GENERAL PRINCIPLES OF MEDICAL RECORD DOCUMENTATION

The principles of documentation listed below are applicable to all types of medical and surgical services in all settings. For Evaluation and Management (E/M) services, the nature and amount of physician work and documentation varies by type of service, place of service and the patient's status. The general principles listed below may be modified to account for these variable circumstances in providing E/M services.

1. The medical record should be complete and legible.

2. The documentation of each patient encounter should include:

    *   reason for encounter and relevant history, physical examination findings, and prior diagnostic test results;

    *   assessment, clinical impression, or diagnosis;

    *   plan for care; and

    *   date and legible identity of the observer.

3. If not documented, the rationale for ordering diagnostic and other ancillary services should be easily inferred.

4. Past and present diagnoses should be accessible to the treating and/or consulting physician.

5. Appropriate health risk factors should be identified.

6. The patient's progress, response to and changes in treatment, and revision of diagnosis should be documented.

7. The CPT and ICD-9-CM codes reported on the health insurance claim form should be supported by the documentation in the medical record.

III. DOCUMENTATION OF E/M SERVICES

This publication provides definitions and documentation guidelines for the three key components of E/M services and for visits which consist predominately of counseling or coordination of care. The three *key* components--history, examination, and medical decision making--appear in the descriptors for office and other outpatient services, hospital observation services, hospital inpatient services, consultations, emergency department services, nursing facility services, domiciliary care services, and home services. While some of the text of CPT has been repeated in this publication, the reader should refer to CPT for the complete descriptors for E/M services and instructions for selecting a level of service. Documentation guidelines are identified by the symbol • DG.

The descriptors for the levels of E/M services recognize seven components which are used in defining the levels of E/M services. These components are:

- history;
- examination;
- medical decision making;
- counseling;
- coordination of care;
- nature of presenting problem; and
- time.

The first three of these components (i.e., history, examination and medical decision making) are the key components in selecting the level of E/M services. In the case of visits which consist predominantly of counseling or coordination of care, time is the key or controlling factor to qualify for a particular level of E/M service.

Because the level of E/M service is dependent on two or three key components, performance and documentation of one component (eg, examination) at the highest level does not necessarily mean that the encounter in its entirety qualifies for the highest level of E/M service.

These Documentation Guidelines for E/M services reflect the needs of the typical adult population. For certain groups of patients, the recorded information may vary slightly from that described here. Specifically, the medical records of infants, children, adolescents and pregnant women may have additional or modified information recorded in each history and examination area.

As an example, newborn records may include under history of the present illness (HPI) the details of mother's pregnancy and the infant's status at birth; social history will focus on family structure; family history will focus on congenital anomalies and hereditary disorders in the family. In addition, the content of a pediatric examination will vary with the age and development of the child. Although not specifically defined in these documentation guidelines, these patient group variations on history and examination are appropriate.

A. DOCUMENTATION OF HISTORY

The levels of E/M services are based on four levels of history (Problem Focused, Expanded Problem Focused, Detailed, and Comprehensive). Each type of history includes some or all of the following elements:

- Chief complaint (CC)

- History of present illness (HPI)

- Review of systems (ROS) and

- Past, family, and/or social history (PFSH).

The extent of the history of present illness, review of systems, and past, family and/or social history that is obtained and documented is dependent upon clinical judgment and the nature of the presenting problem(s).

The chart below shows the progression of the elements required for each type of history. To qualify for a given type of history all three elements in the table must be met. (A chief complaint is indicated at all levels.)

History of Present Illness (HPI)	Review of Systems (ROS)	Past, Family, and/or Social History (PFSH)	Type of History
Brief	N/A	N/A	*Problem Focused*
Brief Problem	Problem Pertinent	N/A	*Focused Expanded Problem*
Extended	Extended	Pertinent	*Detailed*
Extended	Complete	Complete	*Comprehensive*

- *DG: The CC, ROS and PFSH may be listed as separate elements of history, or they may be included in the description of the history of the present illness.*

- *DG: A ROS and/or a PFSH obtained during an earlier encounter does not need to be re-recorded if there is evidence that the physician reviewed and updated the previous information. This may occur when a physician updates his/her own record or in an institutional setting or group practice where many physicians use a common record. The review and update may be documented by:*

  - *describing any new ROS and/or PFSH information or noting there has been no change in the information; and*

  - *noting the date and location of the earlier ROS and/or PFSH.*

- *DG: The ROS and/or PFSH may be recorded by ancillary staff or on a form completed by the patient. To document that the physician reviewed the information, there must be a notation supplementing or confirming the information recorded by others.*

- *DG: If the physician is unable to obtain a history from the patient or other source, the record should describe the patient's condition or other circumstance that precludes obtaining a history.*

Definitions and specific documentation guidelines for each of the elements of history are listed below.

CHIEF COMPLAINT (CC)
The CC is a concise statement describing the symptom, problem, condition, diagnosis, physician recommended return, or other factor that is the reason for the encounter, usually stated in the patient's own words.

- *DG: The medical record should clearly reflect the chief complaint.*

HISTORY OF PRESENT ILLNESS (HPI)

The HPI is a chronological description of the development of the patient's present illness from the first sign and/or symptom or from the previous encounter to the present. It includes the following elements:
- location ,
- quality ,
- severity,
- duration,
- timing,
- context ,
- modifying factors, and
- associated signs and symptoms.

Brief and *extended* HPIs are distinguished by the amount of detail needed to accurately characterize the clinical problem(s).

A *brief* HPI consists of one to three elements of the HPI.
- *DG: The medical record should describe one to three elements of the present illness (HPI).*

An *extended* HPI consists of at least four elements of the HPI or the status of at least three chronic or inactive conditions.
- *DG: The medical record should describe at least four elements of the present illness (HPI), or the status of at least three chronic or inactive conditions.*

REVIEW OF SYSTEMS (ROS)

A ROS is an inventory of body systems obtained through a series of questions seeking to identify signs and/or symptoms that the patient may be experiencing or has experienced.

For purposes of ROS, the following systems are recognized:
- Constitutional Symptoms (eg, fever, weight loss)
- Eyes
- Ears, Nose, Mouth, and Throat
- Cardiovascular
- Respiratory
- Gastrointestinal
- Genitourinary
- Musculoskeletal
- Integumentary (skin and/or breast)
- Neurological
- Psychiatric
- Endocrine
- Hematologic/Lymphatic
- Allergic/Immunologic

A *problem pertinent* ROS inquires about the system directly related to the problem(s) identified in the HPI.

- *DG: The patient's positive responses and pertinent negatives for the system related to the problem should be documented.*

An *extended* ROS inquires about the system directly related to the problem(s) identified in the HPI and a limited number of additional systems.

- *DG: The patient's positive responses and pertinent negatives for two to nine systems should be documented.*

A *complete* ROS inquires about the system(s) directly related to the problem(s) identified in the HPI, *plus* all additional body systems.

- *DG: At least ten organ systems must be reviewed. Those systems with positive or pertinent negative responses must be individually documented. For the remaining systems, a notation indicating all other systems are negative is permissible. In the absence of such a notation, at least ten systems must be individually documented.*

PAST, FAMILY, AND/OR SOCIAL HISTORY (PFSH)

The PFSH consists of a review of three areas:

- past history (the patient's past experiences with illnesses, operations, injuries and treatments);

- family history (a review of medical events in the patient's family, including diseases which maybe hereditary or place the patient at risk); and

- social history (an age appropriate review of past and current activities).

For certain categories of E/M services that include only an interval history, it is not necessary to record information about the PFSH. Those categories are subsequent hospital care, follow-up inpatient consultations and subsequent nursing facility care.

A *pertinent* PFSH is a review of the history area(s) directly related to the problem(s) identified in the HPI.

- *DG: At least one specific item from any of the three history areas must be documented for a pertinent PFSH.*

A *complete* PFSH is a review of two or all three of the PFSH history areas, depending on the category of the E/M service. A review of all three history areas is required for services that by their nature include a comprehensive assessment or reassessment of the patient. A review of two of the three history areas is sufficient for other services.

- *DG: At least one specific item from two of the three history areas must be documented for a complete PFSH for the following categories of E/M services: office or other outpatient services, established patient; emergency department; domiciliary care, established patient; and home care, established patient.*

- *DG: At least one specific item from each of the three history areas must be documented for a complete PFSH for the following categories of E/M services: office or other outpatient services, new patient; hospital observation services; hospital inpatient services, initial care; consultations; comprehensive nursing facility assessments; domiciliary care, new patient; home care, new patient.*

B. DOCUMENTATION OF EXAMINATION

The levels of E/M services are based on four types of examination:

- *Problem Focused* – a limited examination of the affected body area or organ system.

- *Expanded Problem Focused* – a limited examination of the affected body area or organ system and any other symptomatic or related body area(s) or organ system(s).

- *Detailed* – an extended examination of the affected body area(s) or organ system(s) and any other symptomatic or related body area(s) or organ system(s).

- *Comprehensive* – a general multi-system examination, or complete examination of a single organ system and other symptomatic or related body area(s) or organ system(s).

These types of examinations have been defined for general multi-system and the following single organ systems:

- Cardiovascular
- Ears, Nose, Mouth, and Throat
- Eyes
- Genitourinary (Female)
- Genitourinary (Male)
- Hematologic/Lymphatic/Immunologic
- Musculoskeletal
- Neurological
- Psychiatric
- Respiratory
- Skin

A general multi-system examination or a single organ system examination may be performed by any physician, regardless of specialty. The type (general multi-system or single organ system) and content of examination are selected by the examining physician and are based upon clinical judgment, the patient's history, and the nature of the presenting problem(s).

The content and documentation requirements for each type and level of examination are summarized below and described in detail in tables beginning on page 13. In the tables, organ systems and body areas recognized by CPT for purposes of describing examinations are shown in the left column. The content, or individual elements, of the examination pertaining to that body area or organ system are identified by bullets (•) in the right column.

Parenthetical examples "(eg,...)", have been used for clarification and to provide guidance regarding documentation. Documentation for each element must satisfy any numeric requirements (such as "Measurement of *any three of the following seven...*") included in the description of the element. Elements with multiple components but with no specific numeric requirement (such as "Examination of *liver* and *spleen*") require documentation of at least one component. It is possible for a given examination to be expanded beyond what is defined here. When that occurs, findings related to the additional systems and/or areas should be documented.

- *DG: Specific abnormal and relevant negative findings of the examination of the affected or symptomatic body area(s) or organ system(s) should be documented. A notation of "abnormal" without elaboration is insufficient.*

- *DG: Abnormal or unexpected findings of the examination of any asymptomatic body area(s) or organ system(s) should be described.*

- *DG: A brief statement or notation indicating "negative" or "normal" is sufficient to document normal findings related to unaffected area(s) or asymptomatic organ system(s).*

GENERAL MULTI-SYSTEM EXAMINATIONS

General multi-system examinations are described in detail beginning on page 13. To qualify for a given level of multi-system examination, the following content and documentation requirements should be met:

Problem Focused Examination – should include performance and documentation of one to five elements identified by a bullet (•) in one or more organ system(s) or body area(s).

- *Expanded Problem Focused Examination* – should include performance and documentation of at least six elements identified by a bullet (•) in one or more organ system(s) or body area(s).
- *Detailed Examination* – should include at least six organ systems or body areas. For each system/area selected, performance and documentation of at least two elements identified by a bullet (•) is expected. Alternatively, a detailed examination may include performance and documentation of at least twelve elements identified by a bullet (•) in two or more organ systems or body areas.
- *Comprehensive Examination* – should include at least nine organ systems or body areas. For each system/area selected, all elements of the examination identified by a bullet (•) should be performed, unless specific directions limit the content of the examination. For each area/system, documentation of at least two elements identified by a bullet is expected.

SINGLE ORGAN SYSTEM EXAMINATIONS

The single organ system examinations recognized by CPT are described in detail beginning on page 18. Variations among these examinations in the organ systems and body areas identified in the left columns and in the elements of the examinations described in the right columns reflect differing emphases among specialties. To qualify for a given level of single organ system examination, the following content and documentation requirements should be met:

- *Problem Focused Examination* – should include performance and documentation of one to five elements identified by a bullet (•), whether in a box with a shaded or unshaded border.
- *Expanded Problem Focused Examination* – should include performance and documentation of at least six elements identified by a bullet (•), whether in a box with a shaded or unshaded border.
- *Detailed Examination* – examinations other than the eye and psychiatric examinations should include performance and documentation of at least twelve elements identified by a bullet (•), whether in a box with a shaded or unshaded border.

    Eye and psychiatric examinations should include the performance and documentation of at least nine elements identified by a bullet (•), whether in a box with a shaded or unshaded border.

- ***Comprehensive Examination*** – should include performance of all elements identified by a bullet (•), whether in a shaded or unshaded box. Documentation of every element in each box with a shaded border and at least one element in a box with an unshaded border is expected.

CONTENT AND DOCUMENTATION REQUIREMENTS

General Multi-System Examination

System/Body Area	Elements of Examination
Constitutional	Measurement of **any three of the following seven** vital signs: 1) sitting or standing blood pressure, 2) supine blood pressure, 3) pulse rate and regularity, 4) respiration, 5) temperature, 6) height, 7) weight (May be measured and recorded by ancillary staff) General appearance of patient (eg, development, nutrition, body habitus, deformities, attention to grooming)
Eyes	Inspection of conjunctivae and lids Examination of pupils and irises (eg, reaction to light and accommodation, size and symmetry) Ophthalmoscopic examination of optic discs (eg, size, C/D ratio, appearance) and posterior segments (eg, vessel changes, exudates, hemorrhages)
Ears, Nose, Mouth and Throat	External inspection of ears and nose (eg, overall appearance, scars, lesions, masses) Otoscopic examination of external auditory canals and tympanic membranes Assessment of hearing (eg, whispered voice, finger rub, tuning fork) Inspection of nasal mucosa, septum and turbinates Inspection of lips, teeth and gums Examination of oropharynx: oral mucosa, salivary glands, hard and soft palates, tongue, tonsils and posterior pharynx
Neck	Examination of neck (eg, masses, overall appearance, symmetry, tracheal position, crepitus) Examination of thyroid (eg, enlargement, tenderness, mass)

System/Body Area	Elements of Examination
Respiratory	Assessment of respiratory effort (eg, intercostal retractions, use of accessory muscles, diaphragmatic movement)
	Percussion of chest (eg, dullness, flatness, hyperresonance)
	Palpation of chest (eg, tactile fremitus)
	Auscultation of lungs (eg, breath sounds, adventitious sounds, rubs)
Cardiovascular	Palpation of heart (eg, location, size, thrills)
	Auscultation of heart with notation of abnormal sounds and murmurs
	Examination of:
	• carotid arteries (eg, pulse amplitude, bruits)
	• abdominal aorta (eg, size, bruits)
	• femoral arteries (eg, pulse amplitude, bruits)
	• pedal pulses (eg, pulse amplitude)
	• extremities for edema and/or varicosities
Chest (Breasts)	Inspection of breasts (eg, symmetry, nipple discharge)
	Palpation of breasts and axillae (eg, masses or lumps, tenderness)
Gastrointestinal (Abdomen)	Examination of abdomen with notation of presence of masses or tenderness
	Examination of liver and spleen
	Examination for presence or absence of hernia
	Examination (when indicated) of anus, perineum and rectum, including sphincter tone, presence of hemorrhoids, rectal masses
	Obtain stool sample for occult blood test when indicated

System/Body Area	Elements of Examination
Genitourinary	**MALE:**
	Examination of the scrotal contents (eg, hydrocele, spermatocele, tenderness of cord, testicular mass)
	Examination of the penis
	Digital rectal examination of prostate gland (eg, size, symmetry, nodularity, tenderness)
	FEMALE:
	Pelvic examination (with or without specimen collection for smears and cultures), including
	• Examination of external genitalia (eg, general appearance, hair distribution, lesions) and vagina (eg, general appearance, estrogen effect, discharge, lesions, pelvic support, cystocele, rectocele)
	• Examination of urethra (eg, masses, tenderness, scarring)
	• Examination of bladder (eg, fullness, masses, tenderness)
	• Cervix (eg, general appearance, lesions, discharge)
	Uterus (eg, size, contour, position, mobility, tenderness, consistency, descent or support)
	Adnexa/parametria (eg, masses, tenderness, organomegaly, nodularity)
Lymphatic	Palpation of lymph nodes in **two or more** areas: Neck
	Axillae
	Groin
	Other

System/Body Area	Elements of Examination
Musculoskeletal	Examination of gait and station
	Inspection and/or palpation of digits and nails (eg, clubbing, cyanosis, inflammatory conditions, petechiae, ischemia, infections, nodes)
	Examination of joints, bones and muscles of **one or more of the following six** areas: 1) head and neck; 2) spine, ribs and pelvis; 3) right upper extremity; 4) left upper extremity; 5) right lower extremity; and 6) left lower extremity. The examination of a given area includes:
	• Inspection and/or palpation with notation of presence of any misalignment, asymmetry, crepitation, defects, tenderness, masses, effusions
	• Assessment of range of motion with notation of any pain, crepitation or contracture
	• Assessment of stability with notation of any dislocation (luxation), subluxation or laxity
	• Assessment of muscle strength and tone (eg, flaccid, cog wheel, spastic) with notation of any atrophy or abnormal movements
Skin	Inspection of skin and subcutaneous tissue (eg, rashes, lesions, ulcers)
	Palpation of skin and subcutaneous tissue (eg, induration, subcutaneous nodules, tightening)
Neurologic	Test cranial nerves with notation of any deficits
	Examination of deep tendon reflexes with notation of pathological reflexes (eg, Babinski)
	Examination of sensation (eg, by touch, pin, vibration, proprioception)
Psychiatric	Description of patient's judgment and insight
	Brief assessment of mental status including: • orientation to time, place and person • recent and remote memory • mood and affect (eg, depression, anxiety, agitation)

Content and Documentation Requirements

Level of Exam	Perform and Document:
Problem Focused	**One to five** elements identified by a bullet.
Expanded Problem Focused	**At least six** elements identified by a bullet.
Detailed	**At least two** elements identified by a bullet **from each of six areas/systems** OR **at least twelve** elements identified by a bullet **in two or more areas/systems**.
Comprehensive	Perform **all elements** identified by a bullet in **at least nine** organ systems or body areas and document **at least two** elements identified by a bullet **from each of nine areas/systems.**

Cardiovascular Examination

System/Body Area	Elements of Examination
Constitutional	Measurement of **any three of the following seven** vital signs: 1) sitting or standing blood pressure, 2) supine blood pressure, 3) pulse rate and regularity, 4) respiration, 5) temperature, 6) height, 7) weight (May be measured and recorded by ancillary staff) General appearance of patient (eg, development, nutrition, body habitus, deformities, attention to grooming)
Head and Face	
Eyes	Inspection of conjunctivae and lids (eg, xanthelasma)
Ears, Nose, Mouth and Throat	Inspection of teeth, gums and palate Inspection of oral mucosa with notation of presence of pallor or cyanosis
Neck	Examination of jugular veins (eg, distension; a, v or cannon a waves) Examination of thyroid (eg, enlargement, tenderness, mass)
Respiratory	Assessment of respiratory effort (eg, intercostal retractions, use of accessory muscles, diaphragmatic movement) Auscultation of lungs (eg, breath sounds, adventitious sounds, rubs)
Cardiovascular	Palpation of heart (eg, location, size and forcefulness of the point of maximal impact; thrills; lifts; palpable S3 or S4) Auscultation of heart including sounds, abnormal sounds and murmurs Measurement of blood pressure in two or more extremities when indicated (eg, aortic dissection, coarctation) Examination of: • Carotid arteries (eg, waveform, pulse amplitude, bruits, apical-carotid delay) • Abdominal aorta (eg, size, bruits) • Femoral arteries (eg, pulse amplitude, bruits) • Pedal pulses (eg, pulse amplitude) • Extremities for peripheral edema and/or varicosities

System/Body Area	Elements of Examination
Chest (Breasts)	
Gastrointestinal (Abdomen)	Examination of abdomen with notation of presence of masses or tenderness Examination of liver and spleen Obtain stool sample for occult blood from patients who are being considered for thrombolytic or anticoagulant therapy
Genitourinary (Abdomen)	
Lymphatic	
Musculoskeletal	Examination of the back with notation of kyphosis or scoliosis Examination of gait with notation of ability to undergo exercise testing and/or participation in exercise programs Assessment of muscle strength and tone (eg, flaccid, cog wheel, spastic) with notation of any atrophy and abnormal movements
Extremities	Inspection and palpation of digits and nails (eg, clubbing, cyanosis, inflammation, petechiae, ischemia, infections, Osler's nodes)
Skin	Inspection and/or palpation of skin and subcutaneous tissue (eg, stasis dermatitis, ulcers, scars, xanthomas)
Neurological/ Psychiatric	Brief assessment of mental status including • Orientation to time, place and person, • Mood and affect (eg, depression, anxiety, agitation)

Content and Documentation Requirements

Level of Exam	Perform and Document:
Problem Focused	**One to five** elements identified by a bullet.
Expanded Problem Focused	**At least six** elements identified by a bullet.
Detailed	**At least twelve** elements identified by a bullet.
Comprehensive	Perform **all** elements identified by a bullet; document every element in each box with a shaded border and at least one element in each box with an unshaded border.

System/Body Area	Elements of Examination
Constitutional	Measurement of **any three of the following seven** vital signs: 1) sitting or standing blood pressure, 2) supine blood pressure, 3) pulse rate and regularity, 4) respiration, 5) temperature, 6) height, 7) weight (May be measured and recorded by ancillary staff)
	General appearance of patient (eg, development, nutrition, body habitus, deformities, attention to grooming)
	Assessment of ability to communicate (eg, use of sign language or other communication aids) and quality of voice
Head and Face	Inspection of head and face (eg, overall appearance, scars, lesions and masses)
	Palpation and/or percussion of face with notation of presence or absence of sinus tenderness
	Examination of salivary glands
	Assessment of facial strength
Eyes	Test ocular motility including primary gaze alignment
Ears, Nose, Mouth and Throat	Otoscopic examination of external auditory canals and tympanic membranes including pneumo-otoscopy with notation of mobility of membranes Assessment of hearing with tuning forks and clinical speech reception thresholds (eg, whispered voice, finger rub)
	External inspection of ears and nose (eg, overall appearance, scars, lesions and masses)
	Inspection of nasal mucosa, septum and turbinates
	Inspection of lips, teeth and gums
	Examination of oropharynx: oral mucosa, hard and soft palates, tongue, tonsils and posterior pharynx (eg, asymmetry, lesions, hydration of mucosal surfaces)
	Inspection of pharyngeal walls and pyriform sinuses (eg, pooling of saliva, asymmetry, lesions)
	Examination by mirror of larynx including the condition of the epiglottis, false vocal cords, true vocal cords and mobility of larynx (Use of mirror not required in children)
	Examination by mirror of nasopharynx including appearance of the mucosa, adenoids, posterior choanae and eustachian tubes (Use of mirror not required in children)

System/Body Area	Elements of Examination
Neck	Examination of neck (eg, masses, overall appearance, symmetry, tracheal position, crepitus)
	Examination of thyroid (eg, enlargement, tenderness, mass)
Respiratory	Inspection of chest including symmetry, expansion and/or assessment of respiratory effort (eg, intercostal retractions, use of accessory muscles, diaphragmatic movement)
	Auscultation of lungs (eg, breath sounds, adventitious sounds, rubs)
Cardiovascular	Auscultation of heart with notation of abnormal sounds and murmurs
	Examination of peripheral vascular system by observation (eg, swelling, varicosities) and palpation (eg, pulses, temperature, edema, tenderness)
Chest (Breasts)	
Gastrointestinal (Abdomen)	
Genitourinary	
Lymphatic	Palpation of lymph nodes in neck, axillae, groin and/or other location
Musculoskeletal	
Extremities	
Skin	
Neurological/ Psychiatric	Test cranial nerves with notation of any deficits
	Brief assessment of mental status including
	• Orientation to time, place and person,
	• Mood and affect (eg, depression, anxiety, agitation)

Content and Documentation Requirements

Level of Exam	Perform and Document:
Problem Focused	**One to five** elements identified by a bullet.
Expanded Problem Focused	**At least six** elements identified by a bullet.
Detailed	**At least twelve** elements identified by a bullet.
Comprehensive	Perform **all** elements identified by a bullet; document every element in each box with a shaded border and at least one element in each box with an unshaded border.

System/Body Area	Elements of Examination
Constitutional	
Head and Face	
Eyes	Test visual acuity (Does not include determination of refractive error)
	Gross visual field testing by confrontation
	Test ocular motility including primary gaze alignment
	Inspection of bulbar and palpebral conjunctivae
	Examination of ocular adnexae including lids (eg, ptosis or lagophthalmos), lacrimal glands, lacrimal drainage, orbits and preauricular lymph nodes
	Examination of pupils and irises including shape, direct and consensual reaction (afferent pupil), size (eg, anisocoria) and morphology
	Slit lamp examination of the corneas including epithelium, stroma, endothelium, and tear film
	Slit lamp examination of the anterior chambers including depth, cells, and flare
	Slit lamp examination of the lenses including clarity, anterior and posterior capsule, cortex, and nucleus
	Measurement of intraocular pressures (except in children and patients with trauma or infectious disease)
	Ophthalmoscopic examination through dilated pupils (unless contraindicated) of
	• Optic discs including size, C/D ratio, appearance (eg, atrophy, cupping, tumor elevation) and nerve fiber layer
	• Posterior segments including retina and vessels (eg, exudates and hemorrhages)
Ears, Nose, Mouth and Throat	
Neck	
Respiratory	

System/Body Area	Elements of Examination
Cardiovascular	
Chest (Breasts)	
Gastrointestinal (Abdomen)	
Genitourinary	
Lymphatic	
Musculoskeletal	
Extremities	
Skin	
Neurological/ Psychiatric	Brief assessment of mental status including • Orientation to time, place and person • Mood and affect (eg, depression, anxiety, agitation)

Content and Documentation Requirements

Level of Exam	Perform and Document:
Problem Focused	**One to five** elements identified by a bullet.
Expanded Problem Focused	**At least six** elements identified by a bullet.
Detailed	**At least nine** elements identified by a bullet.
Comprehensive	Perform **all** elements identified by a bullet; document every element in each box with a shaded border and at least one element in each box with an unshaded border.

System/Body Area	Elements of Examination
Constitutional	Measurement of **any three of the following seven** vital signs: 1) sitting or standing blood pressure, 2) supine blood pressure, 3) pulse rate and regularity, 4) respiration, 5) temperature, 6) height, 7) weight (May be measured and recorded by ancillary staff) General appearance of patient (eg, development, nutrition, body habitus, deformities, attention to grooming)
Head and Face	
Eyes	
Ears, Nose, Mouth and Throat	
Neck	Examination of neck (eg, masses, overall appearance, symmetry, tracheal position, crepitus) Examination of thyroid (eg, enlargement, tenderness, mass)
Respiratory	Assessment of respiratory effort (eg, intercostal retractions, use of accessory muscles, diaphragmatic movement) Auscultation of lungs (eg, breath sounds, adventitious sounds, rubs)
Cardiovascular	Auscultation of heart with notation of abnormal sounds and murmurs palpation (eg, pulses, temperature, edema, tenderness)
Chest (Breasts)	[See genitourinary (female)]
Gastrointestinal (Abdomen)	Examination of abdomen with notation of presence of masses or tenderness Examination for presence or absence of hernia Examination of liver and spleen Obtain stool sample for occult blood test when indicated

System/Body Area	Elements of Examination
Genitourinary	**MALE:** • Inspection of anus and perineum Examination (with or without specimen collection for smears and cultures) of genitalia including: • Scrotum (eg, lesions, cysts, rashes) • Epididymides (eg, size, symmetry, masses) • Testes (eg, size, symmetry, masses) • Urethral meatus (eg, size, location, lesions, discharge) • Penis (eg, lesions, presence or absence of foreskin, foreskin retractability, plaque, masses, scarring, deformities) Digital rectal examination including: • Prostate gland (eg, size, symmetry, nodularity, tenderness) • Seminal vesicles (eg, symmetry, tenderness, masses, enlargement) • Sphincter tone, presence of hemorrhoids, rectal masses

System/Body Area	Elements of Examination
Genitourinary (Cont'd)	**FEMALE:** Includes **at least seven of the following eleven** elements identified by bullets: • Inspection and palpation of breasts (eg, masses or lumps, tenderness, symmetry, nipple discharge) • Digital rectal examination including sphincter tone, presence of hemorrhoids, rectal masses Pelvic examination (with or without specimen collection for smears and cultures) including: • External genitalia (eg, general appearance, hair distribution, lesions) Urethral meatus (eg, size, location, lesions, prolapse) • Urethra (eg, masses, tenderness, scarring) • Bladder (eg, fullness, masses, tenderness) • Vagina (eg, general appearance, estrogen effect, discharge, lesions, pelvic support, cystocele, rectocele) • Cervix (eg, general appearance, lesions, discharge) • Uterus (eg, size, contour, position, mobility, tenderness, consistency, descent or support) • Adnexa/parametria (eg, masses, tenderness, organomegaly, nodularity) • Anus and perineum
Lymphatic	• Palpation of lymph nodes in neck, axillae, groin and/or other location
Musculoskeletal	
Extremities	
Skin	• Inspection and/or palpation of skin and subcutaneous tissue (eg, rashes, lesions, ulcers)
Neurological/ Psychiatric	Brief assessment of mental status including • Orientation (eg, time, place and person) and • Mood and affect (eg, depression, anxiety, agitation)

Content and Documentation Requirements

Level of Exam	Perform and Document:
Problem Focused	**One to five** elements identified by a bullet.
Expanded Problem Focused	**At least six** elements identified by a bullet.
Detailed	**At least twelve** elements identified by a bullet.
Comprehensive	Perform **all** elements identified by a bullet; document every element in each box with a shaded border and at least one element in each box with an unshaded border.

Hematologic/Lymphatic/Immunologic Examination

System/Body Area	Elements of Examination
Constitutional	Measurement of **any three of the following seven** vital signs: 1) sitting or standing blood pressure, 2) supine blood pressure, 3) pulse rate and regularity, 4) respiration, 5) temperature, 6) height, 7) weight (May be measured and recorded by ancillary staff) General appearance of patient (eg, development, nutrition, body habitus, deformities, attention to grooming)
Head and Face	Palpation and/or percussion of face with notation of presence or absence of sinus tenderness
Eyes	Inspection of conjunctivae and lids
Ears, Nose, Mouth and Throat	Otoscopic examination of external auditory canals and tympanic membranes Inspection of nasal mucosa, septum and turbinates Inspection of teeth and gums Examination of oropharynx (eg, oral mucosa, hard and soft palates, tongue, tonsils, posterior pharynx)
Neck	• Examination of neck (eg, masses, overall appearance, symmetry, tracheal position, crepitus) • Examination of thyroid (eg, enlargement, tenderness, mass)
Respiratory	Assessment of respiratory effort (eg, intercostal retractions, use of accessory muscles, diaphragmatic movement) Auscultation of lungs (eg, breath sounds, adventitious sounds, rubs)
Cardiovascular	Auscultation of heart with notation of abnormal sounds and murmurs Examination of peripheral vascular system by observation (eg, swelling, varicosities) and palpation (pulses, temperature, edema, tenderness)
Chest (Breasts)	
Gastrointestinal (Abdomen)	Examination of abdomen with notation of presence of masses or tenderness Examination of liver and spleen
Genitourinary	

System/Body Area	Elements of Examination
Lymphatic	Palpation of lymph nodes in neck, axillae, groin, and/or other location
Musculoskeletal	
Extremities	Inspection and palpation of digits and nails (eg, clubbing, cyanosis, inflammation, petechiae, ischemia, infections, nodes)
Skin	Inspection and/or palpation of skin and subcutaneous tissue (eg, rashes, lesions, ulcers, ecchymoses, bruises)
Neurological/ Psychiatric	Brief assessment of mental status including • Orientation to time, place and person • Mood and affect (eg, depression, anxiety, agitation)

Content and Documentation Requirements

Level of Exam	Perform and Document:
Problem Focused	**One to five** elements identified by a bullet.
Expanded Problem Focused	**At least six** elements identified by a bullet.
Detailed	**At least twelve** elements identified by a bullet.
Comprehensive	Perform **all** elements identified by a bullet; document every element in each box with a shaded border and at least one element in each box with an unshaded border.

System/Body Area	Elements of Examination
Constitutional	Measurement of **any three of the following seven** vital signs: 1) sitting or standing blood pressure, 2) supine blood pressure, 3) pulse rate and regularity, 4) respiration, 5) temperature, 6) height, 7) weight (May be measured and recorded by ancillary staff)
	General appearance of patient (eg, development, nutrition, body habitus, deformities, attention to grooming)
Head and Face	
Eyes	
Ears, Nose, Mouth and Throat	
Neck	
Respiratory	
Cardiovascular	Examination of peripheral vascular system by observation (eg, swelling, varicosities) and palpation (eg, pulses, temperature, edema, tenderness)
Chest (Breasts)	
Gastrointestinal (Abdomen)	
Genitourinary	
Lymphatic	Palpation of lymph nodes in neck, axillae, groin and/or other location

System/Body Area	Elements of Examination
Musculoskeletal	Examination of gait and station
	Examination of joint(s), bone(s) and muscle(s)/ tendon(s) of **four of the following six** areas: 1) head and neck; 2) spine, ribs and pelvis; 3) right upper extremity; 4) left upper extremity; 5) right lower extremity; and 6) left lower extremity. The examination of a given area includes:
	• Inspection, percussion and/or palpation with notation of any misalignment, asymmetry, crepitation, defects, tenderness, masses or effusions
	• Assessment of range of motion with notation of any pain (eg, straight leg raising), crepitation or contracture
	• Assessment of stability with notation of any dislocation (luxation), subluxation or laxity
	• Assessment of muscle strength and tone (eg, flaccid, cog wheel, spastic) with notation of any atrophy or abnormal movements
	NOTE: For the comprehensive level of examination, all four of the elements identified by a bullet must be performed and documented for each of four anatomic areas. For the three lower levels of examination, each element is counted separately for each body area. For example, assessing range of motion in two extremities constitutes two elements.
Extremities	[See musculoskeletal and skin]
Skin	Inspection and/or palpation of skin and subcutaneous tissue (eg, scars, rashes, lesions, cafe-au-lait spots, ulcers) in **four of the following six** areas: 1) head and neck; 2) trunk; 3) right upper extremity; 4) left upper extremity; 5) right lower extremity; and 6) left lower extremity.
	NOTE: For the comprehensive level, the examination of all four anatomic areas must be performed and documented. For the three lower levels of examination, each body area is counted separately. For example, inspection and/or palpation of the skin and subcutaneous tissue of two extremities constitutes two elements.
Neurological/ Psychiatric	Test coordination (eg, finger/nose, heel/ knee/shin, rapid alternating movements in the upper and lower extremities, evaluation of fine motor coordination in young children)
	Examination of deep tendon reflexes and/or nerve stretch test with notation of pathological reflexes (eg, Babinski)
	Examination of sensation (eg, by touch, pin, vibration, proprioception)
	Brief assessment of mental status including
	• Orientation to time, place and person
	• Mood and affect (eg, depression, anxiety, agitation)

Content and Documentation Requirements

Level of Exam	Perform and Document:
Problem Focused	**One to five** elements identified by a bullet.
Expanded Problem Focused	**At least six** elements identified by a bullet.
Detailed	**At least twelve** elements identified by a bullet.
Comprehensive	Perform **all** elements identified by a bullet; document every element in each box with a shaded border and at least one element in each box with an unshaded border.

System/Body Area	Elements of Examination
Constitutional	Measurement of **any three of the following seven** vital signs: 1) sitting or standing blood pressure, 2) supine blood pressure, 3) pulse rate and regularity, 4) respiration, 5) temperature, 6) height, 7) weight (May be measured and recorded by ancillary staff) General appearance of patient (eg, development, nutrition, body habitus, deformities, attention to grooming)
Head and Face	
Eyes	• Ophthalmoscopic examination of optic discs (eg, size, C/D ratio, appearance) and posterior segments (eg, vessel changes, exudates, hemorrhages)
Ears, Nose, Mouth and Throat	
Neck	
Respiratory	
Cardiovascular	• Examination of carotid arteries (eg, pulse amplitude, bruits) Auscultation of heart with notation of abnormal sounds and murmurs Examination of peripheral vascular system by observation (eg, swelling, varicosities) and palpation (eg, pulses, temperature, edema, tenderness)
Chest (Breasts)	
Gastrointestinal (Abdomen)	
Genitourinary	
Lymphatic	

System/Body Area	Elements of Examination
Musculoskeletal	Examination of gait and station Assessment of motor function including: • Muscle strength in upper and lower extremities • Muscle tone in upper and lower extremities (eg, flaccid, cog wheel, spastic) with notation of any atrophy or abnormal movements (eg, fasciculation, tardive dyskinesia)
Extremities	[See musculoskeletal]
Skin	
Neurological	Evaluation of higher integrative functions including: • Orientation to time, place and person • Recent and remote memory • Attention span and concentration • Language (eg, naming objects, repeating phrases, spontaneous speech) • Fund of knowledge (eg, awareness of current events, past history, vocabulary) Test the following cranial nerves: • 2nd cranial nerve (eg, visual acuity, visual fields, fundi) • 3rd, 4th and 6th cranial nerves (eg, pupils, eye movements) • 5th cranial nerve (eg, facial sensation, corneal reflexes) • 7th cranial nerve (eg, facial symmetry, strength) • 8th cranial nerve (eg, hearing with tuning fork, whispered voice and/or finger rub) • 9th cranial nerve (eg, spontaneous or reflex palate movement) • 11th cranial nerve (eg, shoulder shrug strength) • 12th cranial nerve (eg, tongue protrusion) Examination of sensation (eg, by touch, pin, vibration, proprioception) Examination of deep tendon reflexes in upper and lower extremities with notation of pathological reflexes (eg, Babinski) Test coordination (eg, finger/nose, heel/knee/shin, rapid alternating movements in the upper and lower extremities, evaluation of fine motor coordination in young children)
Psychiatric	

Content and Documentation Requirements

Level of Exam	Perform and Document:
Problem Focused	**One to five** elements identified by a bullet.
Expanded Problem Focused	**At least six** elements identified by a bullet.
Detailed	**At least twelve** elements identified by a bullet.
Comprehensive	Perform **all** elements identified by a bullet; document every element in each box with a shaded border and at least one element in each box with an unshaded border.

System/Body Area	Elements of Examination
Constitutional	Measurement of **any three of the following seven** vital signs: 1) sitting or standing blood pressure, 2) supine blood pressure, 3) pulse rate and regularity, 4) respiration, 5) temperature, 6) height, 7) weight (May be measured and recorded by ancillary staff)
	General appearance of patient (eg, development, nutrition, body habitus, deformities, attention to grooming)
Head and Face	
Eyes	
Ears, Nose, Mouth and Throat	
Neck	
Respiratory	
Cardiovascular	
Chest (Breasts)	
Gastrointestinal (Abdomen)	
Genitourinary	
Lymphatic	
Musculoskeletal	Assessment of muscle strength and tone (eg, flaccid, cog wheel, spastic) with notation of any atrophy and abnormal movements
	Examination of gait and station
Extremities	
Skin	
Neurological	

System/Body Area	Elements of Examination
Psychiatric	

- Description of speech including: rate; volume; articulation; coherence; and spontaneity with notation of abnormalities (eg, perseveration, paucity of language)
- Description of thought processes including: rate of thoughts; content of thoughts (eg, logical vs. illogical, tangential); abstract reasoning; and computation
- Description of associations (eg, loose, tangential, circumstantial, intact)
- Description of abnormal or psychotic thoughts including: hallucinations; delusions; preoccupation with violence; homicidal or suicidal ideation; and obsessions
- Description of the patient's judgment (eg, concerning everyday activities and social situations) and insight (eg, concerning psychiatric condition)

Complete mental status examination including
- Orientation to time, place and person
- Recent and remote memory
- Attention span and concentration
- Language (eg, naming objects, repeating phrases)
- Fund of knowledge (eg, awareness of current events, past history, vocabulary)
- Mood and affect (eg, depression, anxiety, agitation, hypomania, lability)

Content and Documentation Requirements

Level of Exam	Perform and Document:
Problem Focused	**One to five** elements identified by a bullet.
Expanded Problem Focused	**At least six** elements identified by a bullet.
Detailed	**At least nine** elements identified by a bullet.
Comprehensive	Perform **all** elements identified by a bullet; document every element in each box with a shaded border and at least one element in each box with an unshaded border.

Respiratory Examination

System/Body Area	Elements of Examination
Constitutional	Measurement of **any three of the following seven** vital signs: 1) sitting or standing blood pressure, 2) supine blood pressure, 3) pulse rate and regularity, 4) respiration, 5) temperature, 6) height, 7) weight (May be measured and recorded by ancillary staff)
	General appearance of patient (eg, development, nutrition, body habitus, deformities, attention to grooming)
Head and Face	
Eyes	
Ears, Nose, Mouth and Throat	Inspection of nasal mucosa, septum and turbinates
	Inspection of teeth and gums
	Examination of oropharynx (eg, oral mucosa, hard and soft palates, tongue, tonsils and posterior pharynx)
Neck	Examination of neck (eg, masses, overall appearance, symmetry, tracheal position, crepitus)
	Examination of thyroid (eg, enlargement, tenderness, mass)
	Examination of jugular veins (eg, distension; a, v or cannon a waves)
Respiratory	Inspection of chest with notation of symmetry and expansion
	Assessment of respiratory effort (eg, intercostal retractions, use of accessory muscles, diaphragmatic movement)
	Percussion of chest (eg, dullness, flatness, hyperresonance)
	Palpation of chest (eg, tactile fremitus)
	Auscultation of lungs (eg, breath sounds, adventitious sounds, rubs)
Cardiovascular	Auscultation of heart including sounds, abnormal sounds and murmurs
	Examination of peripheral vascular system by observation (eg, swelling, varicosities) and palpation (eg, pulses, temperature, edema, tenderness)
Chest (Breasts)	

System/Body Area	Elements of Examination
Gastrointestinal (Abdomen)	Examination of abdomen with notation of presence of masses or tenderness Examination of liver and spleen
Genitourinary	
Lymphatic	Palpation of lymph nodes in neck, axillae, groin and/or other location
Musculoskeletal	Assessment of muscle strength and tone (eg, flaccid, cog wheel, spastic) with notation of any atrophy and abnormal movements Examination of gait and station
Extremities	Inspection and palpation of digits and nails (eg, clubbing, cyanosis, inflammation, petechiae, ischemia, infections, nodes)
Skin	Inspection and/or palpation of skin and subcutaneous tissue (eg, rashes, lesions, ulcers)
Neurological/ Psychiatric	Brief assessment of mental status including • Orientation to time, place and person • Mood and affect (eg, depression, anxiety, agitation)

Content and Documentation Requirements

Level of Exam	Perform and Document:
Problem Focused	**One to five** elements identified by a bullet.
Expanded Problem Focused	**At least six** elements identified by a bullet.
Detailed	**At least twelve** elements identified by a bullet.
Comprehensive	Perform **all** elements identified by a bullet; document every element in each box with a shaded border and at least one element in each box with an unshaded border.

System/Body Area	Elements of Examination
Constitutional	Measurement of any **three of the following seven** vital signs: 1) sitting or standing blood pressure, 2) supine blood pressure, 3) pulse rate and regularity, 4) respiration, 5) temperature, 6) height, 7) weight (May be measured and recorded by ancillary staff) General appearance of patient (eg, development, nutrition, body habitus, deformities, attention to grooming)
Head and Face	
Eyes	Inspection of conjunctivae and lids
Ears, Nose, Mouth and Throat	Inspection of lips, teeth and gums Examination of oropharynx (eg, oral mucosa, hard and soft palates, tongue, tonsils, posterior pharynx)
Neck	Examination of thyroid (eg, enlargement, tenderness, mass)
Respiratory	
Cardiovascular	Examination of peripheral vascular system by observation (eg, swelling, varicosities) and palpation (eg, pulses, temperature, edema, tenderness)
Chest (Breasts)	
Gastrointestinal (Abdomen)	Examination of liver and spleen Examination of anus for condyloma and other lesions
Genitourinary	
Lymphatic	Palpation of lymph nodes in neck, axillae, groin and/or other location
Musculoskeletal	
Extremities	Inspection and palpation of digits and nails (eg, clubbing, cyanosis, inflammation, petechiae, ischemia, infections, nodes)

Skin Examination

System/Body Area	Elements of Examination
Skin	Palpation of scalp and inspection of hair of scalp, eyebrows, face, chest, pubic area (when indicated) and extremities
	Inspection and/or palpation of skin and subcutaneous tissue (eg, rashes, lesions, ulcers, susceptibility to and presence of photo damage) in **eight of the following ten areas**:
	Head, including the face and Neck Chest, including breasts and axillae Abdomen Genitalia, groin, buttocks Back Right upper extremity Left upper extremity Right lower extremity Left lower extremity
	NOTE: For the comprehensive level, the examination of at least eight anatomic areas must be performed and documented. For the three lower levels of examination, each body area is counted separately. For example, inspection and/or palpation of the skin and subcutaneous tissue of the right upper extremity and the left upper extremity constitutes two elements.
	Inspection of eccrine and apocrine glands of skin and subcutaneous tissue with identification and location of any hyperhidrosis, chromhidroses or bromhidrosis
Neurological/ Psychiatric	Brief assessment of mental status including
	• Orientation to time, place and person
	• Mood and affect (eg, depression, anxiety, agitation)

Content and Documentation Requirements

Level of Exam	Perform and Document:
Problem Focused	**One to five** elements identified by a bullet.
Expanded Problem Focused	**At least six** elements identified by a bullet.
Detailed	**At least twelve** elements identified by a bullet.
Comprehensive	Perform **all** elements identified by a bullet; document every element in each box with a shaded border and at least one element in each box with an unshaded border.

C. DOCUMENTATION OF THE COMPLEXITY OF MEDICAL DECISION MAKING

The levels of E/M services recognize four types of medical decision making (straightforward, low complexity, moderate complexity and high complexity). Medical decision making refers to the complexity of establishing a diagnosis and/or selecting a management option as measured by:

- the number of possible diagnoses and/or the number of management options that must be considered;
- the amount and/or complexity of medical records, diagnostic tests, and/or other information that must be obtained, reviewed and analyzed; and
- the risk of significant complications, morbidity and/or mortality, as well as comorbidities, associated with the patient's presenting problem(s), the diagnostic procedure(s) and/or the possible management options.

The chart below shows the progression of the elements required for each level of medical decision making. To qualify for a given type of decision making, **two of the three elements in the table must be either met or exceeded.**

Number of diagnoses or management options	Amount and/or complexity of data to be reviewed	Risk of complications and/or morbidity or mortality	Type of decision making
Minimal	Minimal or None	Minimal	*Straightforward*
Limited	Limited	Low	*Low Complexity*
Multiple	Moderate	Moderate	*Moderate Complexity*
Extensive	Extensive	High	*High Complexity*

Each of the elements of medical decision making is described below.

NUMBER OF DIAGNOSES OR MANAGEMENT OPTIONS

The number of possible diagnoses and/or the number of management options that must be considered is based on the number and types of problems addressed during the encounter, the complexity of establishing a diagnosis and the management decisions that are made by the physician.

Generally, decision making with respect to a diagnosed problem is easier than that for an identified but undiagnosed problem. The number and type of diagnostic tests employed may be an indicator of the number of possible diagnoses. Problems which are improving or resolving are less complex than those which are worsening or failing to change as expected. The need to seek advice from others is another indicator of complexity of diagnostic or management problems.

> *DG:* *For each encounter, an assessment, clinical impression, or diagnosis should be documented. It may be explicitly stated or implied in documented decisions regarding management plans and/or further evaluation.*

> • *For a presenting problem with an established diagnosis the record should reflect whether the problem is: a) improved, well controlled, resolving or resolved; or, b) inadequately controlled, worsening, or failing to change as expected.*
> • *For a presenting problem without an established diagnosis, the assessment or clinical impression may be stated in the form of differential diagnoses or as a "possible", "probable", or "rule out" (R/O) diagnosis.*

> *DG:* *The initiation of, or changes in, treatment should be documented. Treatment includes a wide range of management options including patient instructions, nursing instructions, therapies, and medications.*

> *DG:* *If referrals are made, consultations requested or advice sought, the record should indicate to whom or where the referral or consultation is made or from whom the advice is requested.*

AMOUNT AND/OR COMPLEXITY OF DATA TO BE REVIEWED

The amount and complexity of data to be reviewed is based on the types of diagnostic testing ordered or reviewed. A decision to obtain and review old medical records and/or obtain history from sources other than the patient increases the amount and complexity of data to be reviewed.

Discussion of contradictory or unexpected test results with the physician who performed or interpreted the test is an indication of the complexity of data being reviewed. On occasion the physician who ordered a test may personally review the image, tracing or specimen to supplement information from the physician who prepared the test report or interpretation; this is another indication of the complexity of data being reviewed.

DG: *If a diagnostic service (test or procedure) is ordered, planned, scheduled, or performed at the time of the E/M encounter, the type of service, eg, lab or x-ray, should be documented.*

DG: *The review of lab, radiology and/or other diagnostic tests should be documented. A simple notation such as "WBC elevated" or "chest x-ray unremarkable" is acceptable. Alternatively, the review may be documented by initialing and dating the report containing the test results.*

DG: *A decision to obtain old records or decision to obtain additional history from the family, caretaker or other source to supplement that obtained from the patient should be documented.*

DG: *Relevant findings from the review of old records, and/or the receipt of additional history from the family, caretaker or other source to supplement that obtained from the patient should be documented. If there is no relevant information beyond that already obtained, that fact should be documented. A notation of "Old records reviewed" or "additional history obtained from family" without elaboration is insufficient.*

DG: *The results of discussion of laboratory, radiology or other diagnostic tests with the physician who performed or interpreted the study should be documented.*

DG: *The direct visualization and independent interpretation of an image, tracing or specimen previously or subsequently interpreted by another physician should be documented.*

RISK OF SIGNIFICANT COMPLICATIONS, MORBIDITY, AND/OR MORTALITY

The risk of significant complications, morbidity, and/or mortality is based on the risks associated with the presenting problem(s), the diagnostic procedure(s), and the possible management options.

> *DG: Comorbidities/underlying diseases or other factors that increase the complexity of medical decision making by increasing the risk of complications, morbidity, and/or mortality should be documented.*

> *DG: If a surgical or invasive diagnostic procedure is ordered, planned or scheduled at the time of the E/M encounter, the type of procedure, eg, laparoscopy, should be documented.*

> *DG: If a surgical or invasive diagnostic procedure is performed at the time of the E/M encounter, the specific procedure should be documented.*

> *DG: The referral for or decision to perform a surgical or invasive diagnostic procedure on an urgent basis should be documented or implied.*

The following table may be used to help determine whether the risk of significant complications, morbidity, and/or mortality is *minimal, low, moderate,* or *high.* Because the determination of risk is complex and not readily quantifiable, the table includes common clinical examples rather than absolute measures of risk. The assessment of risk of the presenting problem(s) is based on the risk related to the disease process anticipated between the present encounter and the next one. The assessment of risk of selecting diagnostic procedures and management options is based on the risk during and immediately following any procedures or treatment. **The highest level of risk in any one category (presenting problem(s), diagnostic procedure(s), or management options) determines the overall risk.**

TABLE OF RISK

Level of Risk	Presenting Problem(s)	Diagnostic Procedure(s) Ordered	Management Options Selected
Minimal	One self-limited or minor problem, eg, cold, insect bite, tinea corporis	Laboratory tests requiring venipuncture Chest x-rays EKG/EEG Urinalysis Ultrasound, eg, echocardiography KOH prep	Rest Gargles Elastic bandages Superficial dressings
Low	Two or more self-limited or minor problems One stable chronic illness, eg, well controlled hypertension, non-insulin dependent diabetes, cataract, BPH Acute uncomplicated illness or injury, eg, cystitis, allergic rhinitis, simple sprain	Physiologic tests not under stress, eg, pulmonary function tests Non-cardiovascular imaging studies with contrast, eg, barium enema Superficial needle biopsies Clinical laboratory tests requiring arterial puncture Skin biopsies	Over-the-counter drugs Minor surgery with no identified risk factors Physical therapy Occupational therapy IV fluids without additives
Moderate	One or more chronic illnesses with mild exacerbation, progression, or side effects of treatment Two or more stable chronic illnesses Undiagnosed new problem with uncertain prognosis, eg, lump in breast Acute illness with systemic symptoms, eg, pyelonephritis, pneumonitis, colitis Acute complicated injury, eg, head injury with brief loss of consciousness	Physiologic tests under stress, eg, cardiac stress test, fetal contraction stress test Diagnostic endoscopies with no identified risk factors Deep needle or incisional biopsy Cardiovascular imaging studies with contrast and no identified risk factors, eg, arteriogram, cardiac catheterization Obtain fluid from body cavity, eg lumbar puncture, thoracentesis, culdocentesis	Minor surgery with identified risk factors Elective major surgery (open, percutaneous or endoscopic) with no identified risk factors Prescription drug management Therapeutic nuclear medicine IV fluids with additives Closed treatment of fracture or dislocation without manipulation
High	One or more chronic illnesses with severe exacerbation, progression, or side effects of treatment Acute or chronic illnesses or injuries that pose a threat to life or bodily function, eg, multiple trauma, acute MI, pulmonary embolus, severe respiratory distress, progressive severe rheumatoid arthritis, psychiatric illness with potential threat to self or others, peritonitis, acute renal failure An abrupt change in neurologic status, eg, seizure, TIA, weakness, sensory loss	Cardiovascular imaging studies with contrast with identified risk factors Cardiac electrophysiological tests Diagnostic Endoscopies with identified risk factors Discography	Elective major surgery (open, percutaneous or endoscopic) with identified risk factors Emergency major surgery (open, percutaneous or endoscopic) Parenteral controlled substances Drug therapy requiring intensive monitoring for toxicity Decision not to resuscitate or to de-escalate care because of poor prognosis

D.   DOCUMENTATION OF AN ENCOUNTER DOMINATED BY COUNSELING OR COORDINATION OF CARE

In the case where counseling and/or coordination of care dominates (more than 50%) of the physician/patient and/or family encounter (face-to-face time in the office or other or outpatient setting, floor/unit time in the hospital or nursing facility), time is considered the key or controlling factor to qualify for a particular level of E/M services.

> ***DG:*** *If the physician elects to report the level of service based on counseling and/or coordination of care, the total length of time of the encounter (face-to-face or floor time, as appropriate) should be documented and the record should describe the counseling and/or activities to coordinate care.*

Appendix E
Other Resources for
Coding Information

American Medical Association <www.ama-assn.org>
Centers for Medicare & Medicaid Services
<www.cms.hhs.gov>
Ingenix <www.ingenix.com>

Appendix F
A Detailed Analysis of Two Coding Methods Summarized in the Introduction

Scenario

110 patients per week (Garfinkel 2005).

Assume: 4 weeks vacation per year.

Therefore, 110 patients per week × 48 weeks per year = 5,280 patients per year.

Assume: all patients seen in office.

Assume: all patients covered by CMS.

Relative Value Units (RVU) and conversion factor according to CMS data for 2004.

99212 = established patient, problem focused history, problem focused examination, straightforward medical decision making = 1.01 RVU

99213 = established patient, expanded problem focused history, expanded problem focused examination, low complexity medical decision making = 1.41 RVU

99204 = new patient, comprehensive history, comprehensive examination, moderate complexity medical decision making = 3.63 RVU

99205 = new patient, comprehensive history, comprehensive examination, high complexity medical decision making = 4.61 RVU

Conversion factor = 37.34 $/RVU

Dr. Average

All patients coded 99213:
5,280 × (1.41 RVU × 37.34 $/RVU) = $277,989.

Dr. Correct

10% of patients coded 99205:
5,280 × 0.1 = 528
528 × (4.61 RVU × 37.34 $/RVU) = $90,889
15% of patients coded 99204:
5,280 × 0.15 = 792
792 × (3.63 RVU × 37.34 $/RVU) = $107,351
55% of patients coded 99213:
5,280 × 0.55 = 2,904
2,904 × (1.41 RVU × 37.34 $/RVU) = $152,894
20% of patients coded 99212:
5,280 × 0.2 = 1,056
1,056 × (1.01 RVU × 37.34 $/RVU) = $39,825
$90,889 + $107,351 + $152,894 + $39,825 = $390,959

Actual average 2004 practice revenue for general practitioners = $260,000 (Lowes 2005).

References

Garfinkel WG. Exclusive survey: Productivity takes a dip. Medical Economics, Nov 18, 2005.

Lowes R. Exclusive survey: The earnings freeze—now it's everybody's problem. Medical Economics, Sep 16, 2005.

Index

American Medical Association
(AMA), 2, 7, 115

Cardiovascular examination, 32, 36,
57, 62, 79–84
CC. *See* Chief complaint
Centers for Medicare and Medicaid
(CMS), 1, 115
  audit liability, 4, 7
  fee schedule, 2
  RVUs and, 7
Chest (breasts), 33, 38
Chief complaint (CC), 71, 72
  low back pain, new patient
consultation template, 61
  patient consultation template, 55
  Step 3, history and physical
examination levels, 25, 28
CMS. *See* Centers for Medicare and
Medicaid
Complications, morbidity, mortality
risks, 17, 18, 112
Constitutional examinations, 16, 30,
31, 37, 57, 62

Consultations
  CPT codes, 10–11
  documentation of, 10–11
Content, documentation
requirements, 79
Counseling, care coordination, 114
CPT. *See* Current Procedural
Terminology coding
Cranial nerves, 58
Current Procedural Terminology
(CPT) coding. *See also* Step
1, patient category; Step 2,
Medical Decision-Making
Table; Step 3, history and
physical examination levels;
Step 4, CTP code and
modifier
  accuracy, 3
  additional resources, 115
  code levels, 2
  coding methods analysis (detailed),
117–118
  coding strategies, 3–4
  consultations, 10–11

121

Current Procedural Terminology
    (CPT) coding. (*cont.*)
  Explanation of Benefits, 7
  history and physical, 6
  modifier identification, 43–48,
    52–53
  patient locations, types, 11–13, 45,
    51
  service levels, 3
  step-by-step approach, 6
  strategies comparison, 4

Data complexity, 111
Deep tendon reflexes, 59, 63
Dictation templates, 5–6, 55–59,
    61–63
Documentation Guidelines for
    Evaluation and Management
    Services (1997), 5
  cardiovascular examination,
    79–84
  CC, 71, 72
  complications, morbidity, mortality
    risks, 112
  comprehensive examination, 79
  content, documentation
    requirements, 79
  counseling, care coordination, 114
  data complexity, 111
  detailed examination, 78
  ear, nose, throat examination,
    86–87
  expanded problem focused, 78
  eye examination, 89–91
  general multi-system examinations,
    77–78, 79–83
  genitourinary examination,
    92–94

  hematologic/lymphatic/
    immunologic examination,
    95–97
  HPI, 5
  medical decision-making,
    complexity documentation,
    109
  musculoskeletal examination,
    98–101
  neurological examination,
    101–103
  number of diagnoses, management
    options, 110
  PFSH, 71, 75–76
  problem focused, 78
  psychiatric examination, 104
  respiratory examination, 105–107
  ROS, 71, 74
  skin examination, 108
  Table of Risk, 113
Drug allergies, 62

E/M. *See* Evaluation and
    Management
E/M Coding Guide, 6, 51–42. *See
    also* CPT coding
Ear, nose, throat examination, 31–32,
    36, 38, 86–87
Electronic Medical Records (EMR),
    5
EMR. *See* Electronic Medical
    Records
Evaluation and Management (E/M),
    2
Explanation of benefits, 7
Extremities, 38
Eye examinations, 30, 31, 36, 38, 57,
    89–91

Gastrointestinal (abdomen) examinations, 33, 38
Genitourinary examination, 33, 38, 62, 92–94

Head, face, 36, 38
Hematologic/lymphatic/immunologic examination, 95–97
Higher integrative functions, 58, 63
History and physical examination, 6, 15
    brief *vs.* extended, 26
    chief complaint, 25, 28
    chronological description, 25–26
    code guide summary, 29
    definition guidelines, 27
    examination categories, 29–35
    general *vs.* single organ system, 37–41
    level selection, 51
    neurological examination, 36–39
    number of items, 25
    pertinent positives, 26
    PFSH, 27–28, 71, 75–76
    problem *vs.* complete system reviews, 26
    recognized body systems, 26
    single organ system examination, 35–36
    system/body area, elements of examination, 30–39
History of present illness (HPI), 5, 71
HPI. *See* History of present illness

Identify patient category, 9–13, 51
Ingenix, 115

Levels of service, 43–44
Location inpatient, 51
    hospital discharge E/M code, 12
    initial, subsequent encounters, 11–12
Low back pain, new patient consultation template
    cardiovascular physical examination, 62
    care plan, 63
    CC, 61
    constitutional physical examination, 62
    deep tendon reflexes, 59, 63
    diagnosis, 63
    drug allergies, 62
    genitourinary, 62
    higher integrative functions, 63
    medications, 62
    musculoskeletal examination, 62–63
    neurological, 62–63
    pin prick, 63
    present illness history, 61
    sensation, 63
    social history, 62
    systems review, 61–62
Lymphatic system, 34, 38, 95–97

Medical decision-making
    care plan, 63
    complexity documentation, 109
    diagnosis, 63
Medical Decision-Making Table, 15–24, 51–52
    CMS guidelines and, 17
    common patient complaints and, 16

Medical Decision-Making Table,
    (*cont.*)
  comorbid conditions, 17
  complexity types, 22–23
  complications, interventions
      comorbidity risks and, 18
  Data Review, 17–18
  degree of complexity
      determination, 16–17
  diagnosis, management options,
      17, 21, 22–23
  history and examination, 15
  patient evaluation order, 16
  sequence, 15
  sub-components, 15–16
  Table of Risk, 18–22, 113
    Diagnostic Procedures Ordered,
        18, 20
    Presenting Problem, 18–19
  terms, 16
Medications, 56, 62
Modifiers, CPT coding, 46–47
Multi-system examinations, 77–78,
    79–83
  cardiovascular, 32
  chest (breasts), 33
  constitutional, 30, 31
  ears, nose, mouth, throat,
      31–32
  eyes, 30, 31
  gastrointestinal (abdomen), 33
  genitourinary, 33
  lymphatic, 34
  musculoskeletal, 34
  neck, 32
  neurological, 35
  psychiatric, 35
  respiratory, 32
  skin, 35

Musculoskeletal examination, 38,
    57–58, 62–63, 98–101

Neck, 32, 36, 38
Neurological examination, 35, 39,
    58, 62–63, 101–103
  cardiovascular, 36, 57
  chest (breasts), 38
  constitutional, 36, 37, 57
  coordination, 59
  cranial nerves, 58
  deep tendon reflexes, 59, 63
  dictation template
    care plan, 59
    CC, 55
    diagnosis, 59
    drug allergies, 56
    family history, 56
    medications, 56
    past history, 56
    present illness history, 56
    social history, 56
    systems review, 56
  ears, nose, mouth, throat, 36,
      38
  extremities, 38
  eyes, 36, 38, 57
  gastrointestinal (abdomen), 38
  genitourinary, 38
  head, face, 36, 38
  higher integrative functions
      evaluation, 58
  lymphatic, 38
  musculoskeletal, 38, 57–58
  neck, 36, 38
  pin prick, 58–59
  psychiatric, 39
  respiratory, 36, 38
  sensation, 58

Number of diagnoses, management options, 110

Office or other outpatient services
    confirmatory consultation, 10
    consultation, 10
    established, 10
    new, 10
Outpatient category, 10, 51

Past, family, and/or social history
        (PFSH), 27–28, 56, 62, 71,
        75–76. *See also* Patient
        history
Patient category, 9–13, 12, 51. *See
        also* Step 1, patient category
Patient consultation template,
        55–59
Patient encounter, documentation of,
        5
Patient history, 27–28
    comprehensive, 27–28
    detailed, 28
    expanded problem, 28
    problem focused, 28
PFSH. *See* Past, family, and/or social
        history
Physician fee schedule services,
        dollar amount spent on, 3
Pin prick, 58–59, 63
Psychiatric examination, 35, 39,
        104

Reimbursement rates, 1–2
Relative Value Units (RVU), 7,
        46
Respiratory examination, 32, 36, 38,
        105–107
Review of systems, 71, 74

ROS. *See* Review of systems
RVU. *See* Relative Value Units

Sensation, 58, 63
Skin examination, 35, 108
Step 1, patient category
    CATEGORY, LOCATION and
        TYPE codes, 12, 51
    identify patient category, 9–13,
        51
    location inpatient, 11–13, 51
        hospital discharge E/M code, 12
        initial, subsequent encounters,
            11–12
    office or other outpatient services
        confirmatory consultation, 10
        consultation, 10
        established, 10
        new, 10
Step 2, Medical Decision-Making
        Table, 15–24, 51–52
    CMS guidelines and, 17
    CMS Table of Risk, 18–22
    common patient complaints and,
        16
    comorbid conditions, 17
    complexity types, 22–23
    complications, interventions
        comorbidity risks and, 18
    Data Review, 17–18
    degree of complexity
        determination, 16–17
    diagnosis, management options,
        17, 21, 22–23
    history and examination, 15
    patient evaluation order, 16
    sequence, 15
    subcomponents, 15–16
    Table of Risk, 18–22, 113

Step 2, Medical Decision-Making
     Table, (*cont.*)
   Diagnostic Procedures Ordered,
     18, 20
   Presenting Problem, 18–19
   terms, 16
Step 3, history and physical
     examination levels, 51
   brief *vs.* extended, 26
   chief complaint, 25, 28
   chronological description, 25–26
   CMS definition guidelines, 27
   CMS examination categories,
     29–35
   CMS recognized body systems, 26
   code guide summary, 29
   general *vs.* single organ system,
     37–42

   neurological examination, 36–39
   number of items, 25
   past medical, family, social
     histories, 27–28
   pertinent positives, 26
   problem *vs.* complete system
     reviews, 26
   single organ system examination,
     35–36
   system/body area, elements of
     examination, 30–39
Step 4, CPT code and modifier
   identification, 43–48, 52–53
   levels of service, 43–44
   modifiers, 46–47
   RVU conversion, 46

Table of Risk, 18–22, 113